Pharmaceuticals AND THE Sea

EDITED BY:

Charles W. Jefford
Department of Organic Chemistry
University of Geneva
Geneva, Switzerland

Kenneth L. Rinehart
Roger Adams Laboratory
University of Illinois
Urbana, Illinois, U.S.A.

Lois S. Shield
Roger Adams Laboratory
University of Illinois
Urbana, Illinois, U.S.A.

TECHNOMIC PUBLISHING CO., INC.
LANCASTER · BASEL

Published in the Western Hemisphere by
Technomic Publishing Company, Inc.
851 New Holland Avenue
Box 3535
Lancaster, Pennsylvania 17604 U.S.A.

Distributed in the Rest of the World by
Technomic Publishing AG

Printed in the United States of America
10 9 8 7 6 5 4 3 2 1

Main entry under title:
Pharmaceuticals And The Sea

A Technomic Publishing Company book
Bibliography: p.

Library of Congress Card No. 87-51603
ISBN No. 87762-581-6

Preface

On March 10, 1984, President Ronald Reagan proclaimed the period July 1, 1984 through June 30, 1985, as the "Year of the Ocean". The objectives were to celebrate the anniversary of the creation of an exclusive economic zone encompassing all resources lying within the limit 200 miles off the shores of the USA, and at the same time to render the American public aware of the potential of those marine sources. Earlier, a group of interested private individuals, in anticipation of this occasion, established the Year of the Ocean Foundation. Its mandate was to implement the necessary programs to publicize the importance of the ocean not only from the point of view of conservation, but also as a new frontier to be pioneered. One of the Foundation's basic programs was the sponsoring of the Edwin B. Forsythe Round-Table Conferences. Eight conferences were planned, each would convene experts to speak on what the future holds for the development of the ocean's resources. Consequently, the Year of the Ocean Foundation together with Harbor Branch Foundation, Inc., in conjunction with SeaPharm, Inc., co-sponsored the 8th and final conference on the theme "Pharmaceuticals and the Sea" which took place on October 24-25, 1985, at the Harbor Branch Foundation research facilities in Fort Pierce, Florida. The conference consisted of presentations made by 17 prominent panelists drawn from the USA, Italy and Japan representing academia, industry and Federal agencies. The panelists were invited for their special interest in pharmaceutical and bio-active substances. Participants at the conference came mostly from the USA, but many came from countries abroad having traditional associations with the sea such as New Zealand, Australia, Italy and Japan.

The topics covered ranged from an examination of the degree of success in discovering new drugs from the sea (Section I), through the need for new pharmaceuticals, in particular those that might be found in the sea (Section II), the status of research on marine bio-active compounds (Section III), new isolation and analytical techniques (Section IV), to what is perhaps the most important topic, namely how all these endeavors might be funded (Section V).

The text of these presentations is now compiled in this book which we hope will be a useful compendium. The different perspectives seen by proponents in universities, pharmaceutical companies, Federal funding and regulatory agencies together with a venture capitalist's view, provide, we believe, a valuable commentary on the future of marine pharmaceuticals.

We would like to thank J. Seward Johnson, Jr., President of Harbor Branch Foundation, for graciously hosting the conference. We are also greatly appreciative of the efforts made by the staff at Harbor Branch Foundation. Similarly the staff at the SeaPharm, Inc., offices are to be thanked for coping with the logistics of the conference, especially in dealing with the travel arrangements of the participants. We owe special thanks to Alexander Zaslona for editing and preparing the manuscript for publication. We thank John Boukouvalas for his help in assembling and preparing the numerous diagrams. Lastly we express our gratitude to Marlène Wyss who typed the entire manuscript in her usual impeccable style.

Geneva, Switzerland
Urbana, Illinois

Charles W. Jefford
Kenneth L. Rinehart
Lois S. Shield

Table of Contents

Section I

Past Experience with Marine Sources

Kenneth L. Rinehart
Roger Adams Laboratory, University of Illinois at Urbana-Champaign, Urbana, Illinois 61801, U.S.A.

Successes and Failures of Previous Efforts to Develop New Drug Leads from the Sea

The title assigned to Dr. Brossi and me, "Successes and Failures of Previous Efforts to Develop New Drug Leads from the Sea" implies, correctly, the existence of both. Little systematic effort was applied to the development of marine-derived pharmaceuticals ("drugs from the sea") before 1960, but in the following decade serious attempts were mounted in that direction. By 1968, the field was sufficiently advanced to launch a roughly biennial conference on marine-derived pharmaceuticals, which continued through 1978.[1-5] In addition to the proceedings of these conferences, a number of books appeared during this period on the general subject of marine toxins and other bioactive compounds of marine origin.[6-8] Marine natural products have also been treated in many reviews of a more general nature.[9,10]

PROBLEMS INHERENT IN MARINE COLLECTIONS

After 1979, however, considerable doubt emerged regarding the future of marine pharmaceuticals. The proceedings of the fifth and last Food-Drugs from the Sea Conference, held in 1977, were published with the sub-title "Myth or Reality?". A once promising field had lost some of its lustre and one can ask, "Why has it been difficult to produce a successful marine-derived drug?". The several answers to this question appear to this observer to fall into the three categories which follow: (1) Unfamiliar Territory, (2) Collection and Storage of Samples, and (3) Assays and Isolation.

Unfamiliar Territory. Compounds derived from marine macroorganisms are a novelty on the pharmaceutical scene. At present there are no marine-derived compounds among the pharmaceuticals commercially available in the United States although some marine natural products, e.g., a horseshoe crab extract,[11] are in use as diagnostic agents, and cephalosporin was originally isolated from a *Cephalosporium* species from the Mediterranean.[12] This is a new field. No extensive folklore, such as that which has evolved concerning terrestrial plants,[13-15] is associated with marine species, and in Western civilization there is no tradition for the use of marine materials to relieve human suffering. This contrast was noted ten years ago by Ruggieri,[16] who also observed that while the Romans had certain superstitions about marine species there was no folklore about cures. An exception to this lack of marine folklore lies in the Oriental experience, which differs markedly from the Western avoidance of marine-derived remedies; in Japan and China a number of medicinal properties have been attributed, for example, to seaweeds. (A recent paper also noted the use of seaweed remedies by the San Blas

Indians in Panama.[17]) Nevertheless, only a few entries in the most recent "Dictionary of Chinese Medicine" relate to marine-derived natural products.[18]

Marine toxins represent a second exception to the general lack of marine experience. Primitive peoples may have known little about the curative value of marine species, but they certainly knew about toxins. They knew, for example, that some puffer fish were toxic and that other fish and mussels could be toxic at certain times of the year. Marine toxins have been extensively described by Halstead.[19] It is not surprising that some of the most important uses of marine natural products involve applications of toxins, especially tetrodotoxin,[20] as biological or diagnostic agents.

The obvious reason for this absence of marine folklore is the fact that the ocean is, after all, not man's normal habitat; and below the intertidal zone it is a most unnatural, and can be an unfriendly, environment for him.

Collection and Storage of Samples. Obtaining useful drugs from the sea involves the collection and storage of samples. Since collectors did not know at the outset which species might provide useful drugs, their chances for success depended on the number of samples collected and on statistics. The number of samples collected can obviously be increased by investigations at a variety of both depths and locations. Most early collections were from the intertidal zone. Although the sublittoral zone (surface to -180 feet) has been studied sporadically for some 2000 years with cumbersome equipment (open diving bells, apparently first used by the Greeks, and hard hat diving suits, developed nearly a century ago), a real stimulus to sublittoral research came in the late 1940's with the introduction of SCUBA (self-contained underwater breathing apparatus) and with the work of Cousteau. SCUBA techniques allow freely moving divers, breathing air, to collect samples routinely at -120 feet and, for short periods of time, as deep as -200 feet; using lockout diving procedures and mixed gases to reduce the danger of decompression sickness and nitrogen narcosis,[21] divers may reach greater depths. An added stimulus to underwater research has been the more recent introduction of small submersibles, not only for investigating the deep water environment by means of camera and video, but also for collecting and storing specimens, either by on-board scientists or by remote control. Sample collections by manned submersibles are possible at nearly -3000 feet using Plexiglass bubbles or, with greater difficulty, at perhaps -15,000 feet using metal cylinders with glass portals.[22]

Increasing the depth range of collections enhances considerably the possibility of finding new pharmaceutical agents. This can be illustrated by the results of a recent SeaPharm expedition during which samples were collected by submersible from 100 to 2700 feet below the surface, as well as by SCUBA and snorkeling at shallower depths (Table I).[23]

Most pre-1970 marine collections were limited geographically to the species found during collections near shore-based marine stations. A research vessel, by contrast, can provide transportation to deeper waters and to off-shore or remote locations. It can also provide accompanying laboratory facilities. For investigators not associated with marine institutions, however, ship time is difficult to obtain. From 1972, the National Science Foundation made available to biologists and chemists throughout the U.S., on a research grant basis, the *R/V Alpha Helix*, a ship designed for biological and chemical work near shore at remote sites.[24] The NSF program did much to encourage research on bioactive marine compounds but, unfortunately, the *Alpha Helix* was removed from this valuable duty after about six years.

Table I. % ACTIVITY AT VARIOUS DEPTHS

	% Active (# samples)			
Depth	HSV[a]	CV-1[a]	*E.c.*[a]	*P.a.*[a]
0- 10	10 (20)	39 (28)	9 (81)	0 (81)
10- 100	0 (4)	8 (14)	19 (57)	14 (57)
100- 400	14 (49)	31 (94)	20 (158)	14 (159)
401-1000	12 (86)	21 (68)	15 (101)	11 (101)
1000-1500	8 (26)	23 (84)	7 (88)	3 (88)
1500-2000			0 (9)	0 (9)

[a]HSV = *Herpes simplex*, type 1 (+++, ++, or +/-); CV-1 = *Vesicular stomatitis*-infected monkey kidney cells, complete kill, 16 mm well; *E.c.* = *Escherichia coli*; *P.a.* = *Penicillium atrovenetum*.

I have commented on the statistical desirability of investigating as large a number and variety of species as possible, and additional advocacy of a statistical approach to marine collections is provided later in this volume by Dr. Boyd. Unfortunately, the chance of identifying a useful marine pharmaceutical agent was statistically reduced in several marine programs by restricting collections to the most abundant species found, even though the less abundant and scarce species far outnumber the abundant ones.

Another obstacle to the discovery of bioactivity arose from inappropriate sample storage in early efforts. Specimens were often simply sun-dried, leading, in a tropical climate, to both biological and photochemical degradation. A second method, storing the specimens in alcohol, offered some improvement, since the alcohol halted biological degradation; on the other hand, alcohol reacts with many compounds, producing chemical modification or degradation. There are even reports of the use of the highly reactive formalin as a storage solvent. More modern methods involve either freezing or freeze-drying and, while they may not be completely satisfactory, they reduce sample degradation.

<u>Assays and Isolation</u>. In the early days of marine natural product research, assays to identify pharmacologically active species were often conducted in laboratories hundreds or even thousands of miles from the site of collection. Since the collectors did not know which samples would ultimately prove active, they collected relatively large samples of all specimens and many of them proved to be inactive. Moreover, decomposition often occurred en route to the laboratory.

On-site bioassays solve both problems. Fresh samples are tested, and the collectors can then concentrate on those samples which show the desired activity. It is possible to carry out a variety of on-site assays both on shipboard and in more primitive shore-based laboratories. This ability was demonstrated first in the University of Illinois's 1974 Alpha Helix Baja Expedition[25] and expanded in our 1978 Alpha Helix Caribbean Expedition[26] and in expeditions employing a mobile home or truck as a laboratory, as shown in Table II. On-site assays have been further expanded at SeaPharm, as noted in Mr. Torres's presentation.

Table II. SUCCESSFUL ON-SITE BIOASSAYS[a]

Antimicrobial
Bacillus subtilis, Escherichia coli,
Saccharomyces cerevisiae, Penicillium atrovenetum
Antiviral[b]
HSV-1
VSV
Cytotoxicity[b]
CV-1
L1210[c]
P388[c]
BIA[b]
Frog heart
Immunoregulatory[c]
T-cell mitogenesis
B-cell mitogenesis
MLR[d]

[a]Shipboard and/or mobile lab, University of Illinois expeditions, except as noted. [b]HSV-1 = *Herpes simples* virus, type 1; VSV = vesicular stomatitis virus; CV-1 = monkey kidney cells; BIA = biochemical induction assay. [c]SeaPharm expeditions. [d]Mixed lymphocyte reaction.

In addition to the problems associated with distance, early attempts to obtain marine pharmaceuticals were often hampered by a reliance on *in vivo* bioassays, which required relatively large samples and limited testing to the most abundant species. Finally, descriptions of biological activity were often non-quantitative. As we noted in a 1978 review,[27] many early reports of biological activity, especially antibacterial activity, did not specify concentrations or amounts required to achieve specific effects.

When a desirable bioactivity had been identified, isolation of the compound responsible posed another problem. The long time lapse between submission of a sample and receipt of *in vivo* data made it impractical to follow separation or isolation procedures by bioassay. Even when a quick *in vitro* assay was available, quantitation was often neglected. Most of the early work appears to have been chemistry driven, with isolations restricted to or concentrated on those compounds which were either most abundant or happened to crystallize from solution. There is, of course, no assurance that the most abundant or most crystalline compound will be the most active. Examples abound, but an illustration of this point is the compound plakortin, which was reported as the antimicrobial compound form a *Plakortis* (sponge) species.[28] Plakortin, the methyl ester, is the most abundant compound, but it is orders of magnitude less active as an antifungal agent than the free acid, plakortic acid (Table III).[29]

Table III. ANTIMICROBIAL ACTIVITY

	Zone of Inhibition, mm[a]			
Compound	*B.s.*	*E.c.*	*S.c.*	*P.a.*
Plakortic acid[b]	23	-	40+	34
Plakortin[c]	-(tr)[d]	-	-	-

[a]*B.s.* = *Bacillus subtilis; E.c.* = *Escherichia coli; S.c.* = *Saccharomyces cerevisiae; P.a.* = *Penicillium atrovenetum.* [b]100 μg/disk. [c]1000 μg/disk. [d](tr) indicates trace of activity at 10,000 μg/disk.

BRIEF HISTORICAL PERSPECTIVES

Following those initial comments on problems inherent in early marine pharmaceutical research, I shall review some successes and failures of relatively extensive efforts in specific therapeutic areas: antimicrobial, antitumor, antiviral, and cardioregulatory.

Antimicrobial Activity. The first extensive efforts to find antimicrobial compounds in marine species appear to have been those of Nigrelli and his colleagues at the New York Aquarium, as reviewed in 1960.[30] A contemporary effort was that of Burkholder, one of the discoverers of chloramphenicol, first at the University of Puerto Rico and later at Columbia's Lamont-Doherty Geophysical Laboratory, as reviewed in 1968.[31] Other early efforts included those at Lederle under Webb and, somewhat later, our own extensive surveys in Baja California in 1974[25] and in the Caribbean in 1978.[26] Antimicrobial compounds from marine sources have been reviewed earlier.[27,32] As noted above, many studies were relatively non-quantitative[27] in that they did not include a minimum inhibitory concentration or zone of inhibition, perhaps for good reason; when compared on a quantitative basis with clinically useful antibiotics from terrestrial microorganisms, most marine compounds simply could not measure up to those heavyweight wonder drugs.

Antitumor Activity. Perhaps the most extensive systematic effort of all was the contract program of the National Cancer Institute, directed for over a decade toward the discovery of antitumor agents in marine species. An *in vivo* P388 assay and an *in vitro* KB assay were used in this program to identify a number of very promising species. The results of the program were reviewed at regular intervals by the contractors,[33,34] who concluded that a relatively high incidence of antitumor activity was observable in marine species. Hindrances to developing a drug in the NCI program appear to have been a reliance on a remote *in vivo* assay to identify active extracts and follow separation of bioactive compounds and, perhaps to a lesser degree, storage of samples in alcohol in the field. The NCI program, both in its earlier form and a planned revision, is described more extensively in Dr. Boyd's presentation.

Antitumor compounds from marine sources have been extensively reviewed in a number of volumes devoted to antitumor agents from natural sources.[35,36] At the present time, however, only one marine-derived compound, didemnin B (to be discussed below),[37] has reached clinical trials, although at least two others: dolastatin[38] (whose structure is at present uncertain)[39] and ecteinascidin (whose structure has not been reported)[40,41] appear to be promising candidates.

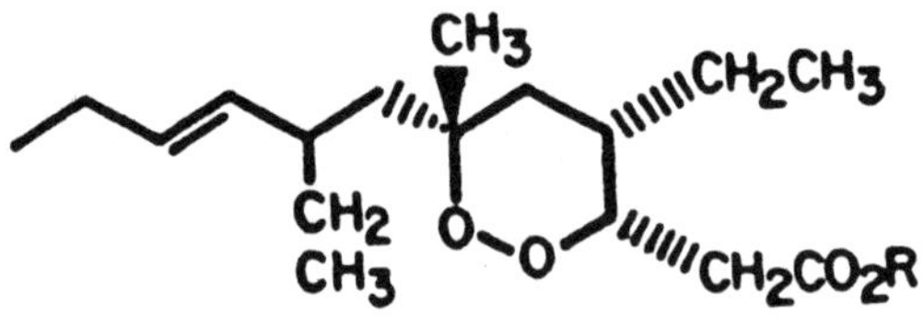

Plakortic Acid: R = H
Plakortin: R = CH_3

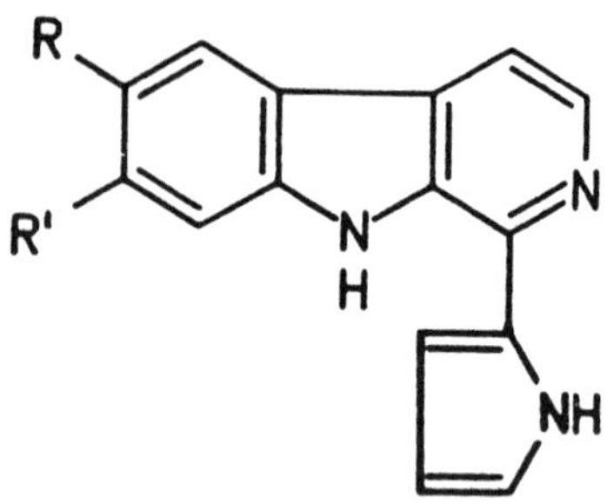

	R	R'
1 (A) :	OH	Br
13 (M) :	OH	H

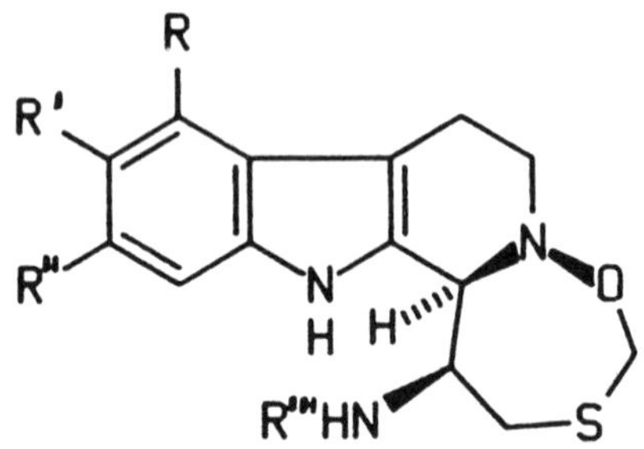

	R	R'	R''	R'''
3 (C) :	H	OH	Br	H
5 (E) :	Br	OH	H	H
6 (F) :	H	OH	Br	$C_2H_3O_2$
11 (K) :	H	H	Br	H
12 (L) :	H	Br	H	H

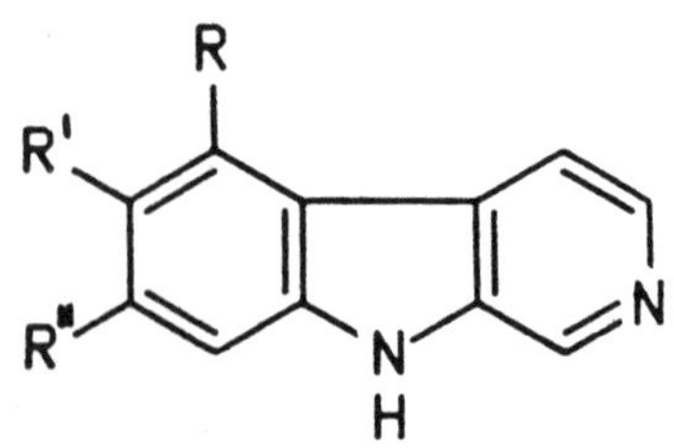

	R	R'	R''
4 (D) :	Br	OH	H
10 (J) :	H	OH	Br
14 (N) :	H	Br	H
15 (O) :	H	H	Br

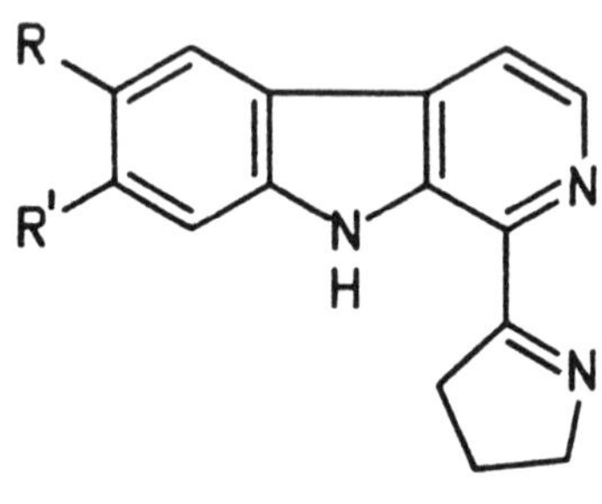

	R	R'
7 (G) :	H	Br
8 (H) :	Br	H
9 (I) :	H	H
16 (P) :	OH	Br
17 (Q) :	OH	H

Scheme I. Structures of the Eudistomins.

	Ile / Val (A.S.)		10	
A.S.	Gly- Ile/Val	Pro	Cys-Leu-Asp-Ser-Asp-Ser-Asp-Gly-Pro-Ser-Val-Arg-Gly-	
A.X.	Gly-Val	Ser	Cys-Leu-Asp-Ser-Asp-Ser-Asp-Gly-Pro-Ser-Val-Arg-Gly-	

	20				30	
A.S.	Asn-Thr-Leu-Ser-Gly	Ile-Ile	Trp-Leu	--------Ala	Gly-Cys-Pro-	
A.X.	Asn-Thr-Leu-Ser-Gly	Thr-Leu	Trp-Leu	Tyr-Pro-Ser	Gly-Cys-Pro-	

			40
A.S.	Ser-Gly-Trp-His-Asp-Cys-Lys	Lys	His-Gly-Pro-Thr-Ile-Gly-Trp-
A.X.	Ser-Gly-Trp-His-Asp-Cys-Lys	Ala	His-Gly-Pro-Thr-Ile-Gly-Trp-

	49
A.S.	Cys-Cys-Lys-Gln
A.X.	Cys-Cys-Lys-Gln

Scheme II. Structures of Sea Anemone Toxins - *Anemonia sulcata* toxin II (A.S.) and *Anthopleura xanthogrammatica* heart stimulant, anthopleurin A (A.X.), with identical residues in boxes.

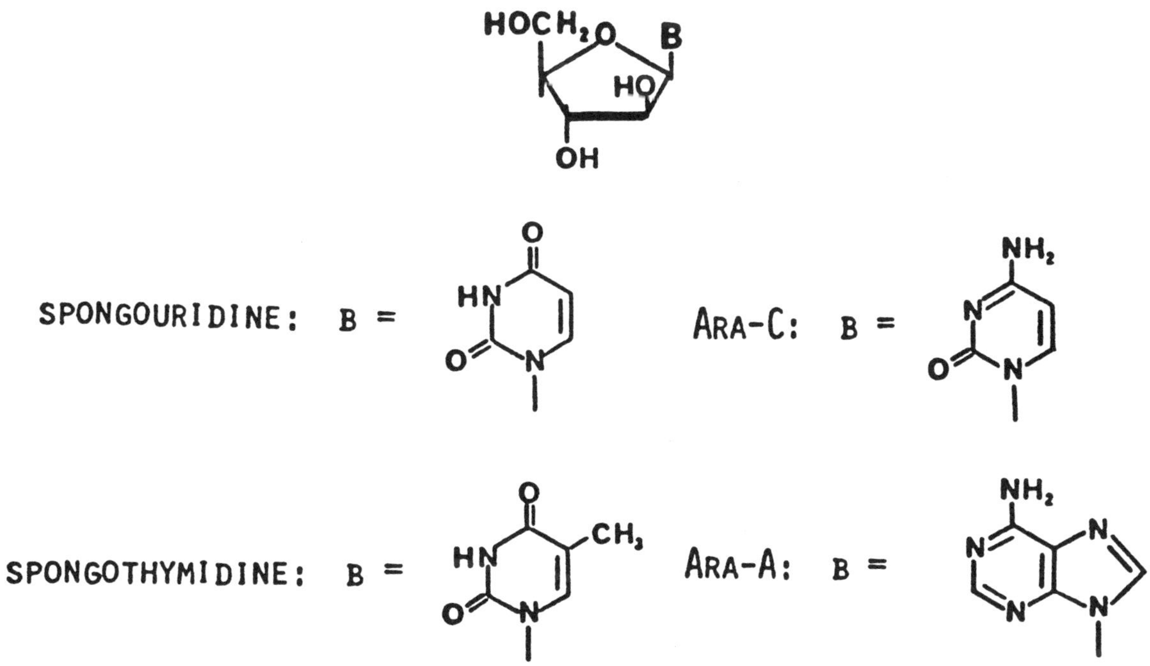

Scheme III. Structures of sponge nucleosides and related arabinosides, Ara-A and Ara-C.

Antiviral Activity. The first systematic investigation of antiviral properties of marine natural products seems to have been that of our 1978 Alpha Helix Caribbean Expedition,[26] during which 650 species (>1350 samples) were assayed for inhibition of *Herpes simplex* virus, type 1. A surprising number of those samples (*ca.* 90) demonstrated antiviral properties, surprising in view of the then prevailing opinion that antiviral activity was a relatively rare property of organic compounds. The antiviral assays carried out on shipboard in a mammalian cell line (monkey kidney, CV−1 cells) also provided an indication of mammalian cytotoxicity, a potential predictor of antitumor activity. An interesting aspect of the study was the observation that the tunicate *Eudistoma olivaceum* provided in the field the most antiviral extract of any species, but that this extract proved inactive when subjected to secondary antiviral testing at the Upjohn Company. To test our hypothesis that the active compound(s) had decomposed, a search was undertaken, the tunicate was re-located in mangrove swamps, and fresh samples were obtained which, indeed, proved to be highly antiviral. Had one relied on remote assays in this case, the activity might never have been detected. Seventeen compounds have now been isolated from that tunicate (see structures in Scheme I)[42] and eudistomins C and E have proved to be especially potent *in vitro* against *Herpes simplex* virus, types 1 and 2. The other potent antiviral agents discovered in that 1978 survey,[26] the didemnins, will be discussed below.

Cardioregulatory Activity. No large-scale systematic search for cardioregulatory activity seems to have been undertaken, but a number of cardioactive compounds have been described, as reviewed elsewhere.[43] The most promising cardioregulators appear to be derived from sea anemones. It has been known for some time that sea anemones produce toxic compounds and further investigation demonstrated that the compounds from some sea anemones are quite active as cardiostimulants. These include the anthopleurins, from *Anthopleura xanthogrammatica*, discovered by Norton at the University of Hawaii,[44] and the ATX toxins from *Anemonia sulcata*, discovered by Beress at the University of Kiel.[45] These are polypeptides of varying chain lengths, and an interesting feature is the very high degree of homology found in the peptides from the different sea anemones (see structures in Scheme II). The utility of the sea anemone cardiostimulants as therapeutic agents has not been established, but they, or some simpler analogues, may be valuable in light of the very narrow therapeutic index of their competitor, digitalis.

Multiple Targets. In addition to the efforts focused on specific therapeutic areas, several pharmaceutical companies or institutes have directed their attentions toward a multiplicity of disease states. These include the Suntory Institute for Biomedical Research, the Roche Institute of Marine Pharmacology, the Mitsubishi-Kasei Institute, and SeaPharm, Inc. The first of these was reviewed elsewhere recently,[47] and the other three will be described in later presentations of this Roundtable.

EXAMPLES OF DRUG LEADS FROM MARINE SOURCES

In this final section I should like to present three examples of leading marine-derived drug candidates past and present with comments on their discovery and ultimate fate.

Ara-C and Ara-A. Cytosine arabinoside (Ara-C) and adenosine arabinoside (Ara-A) are probably the best examples of successful pharmaceutical agents based on marine sources. A significant point is that the compounds isolated in nature were not the drugs named above but two related compounds, thymine arabinoside (spongothymidine) and uracil arabinoside (spongouridine), which were isolated, along with spongosine (2−methoxyadenosine), when they crystallized from the acetone extract of the sponge *Tethya crypta (Cryptotethya crypta)*.[47] A second point is that Bergmann and his collaborators were not looking for nucleosides at all but for steroids from sponges; the nucleosides represented a serendipitous discovery.

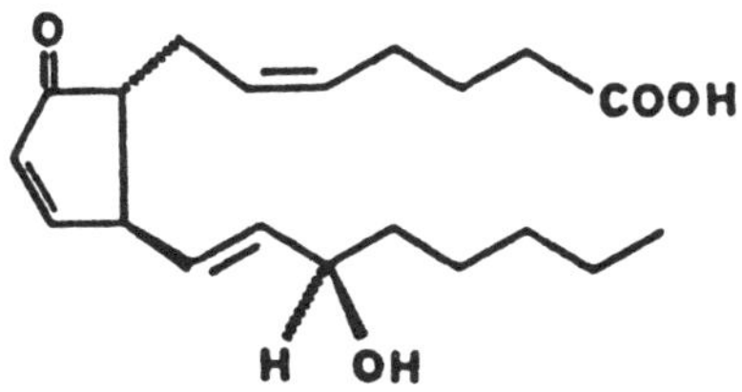

15-*epi*-PGA_2

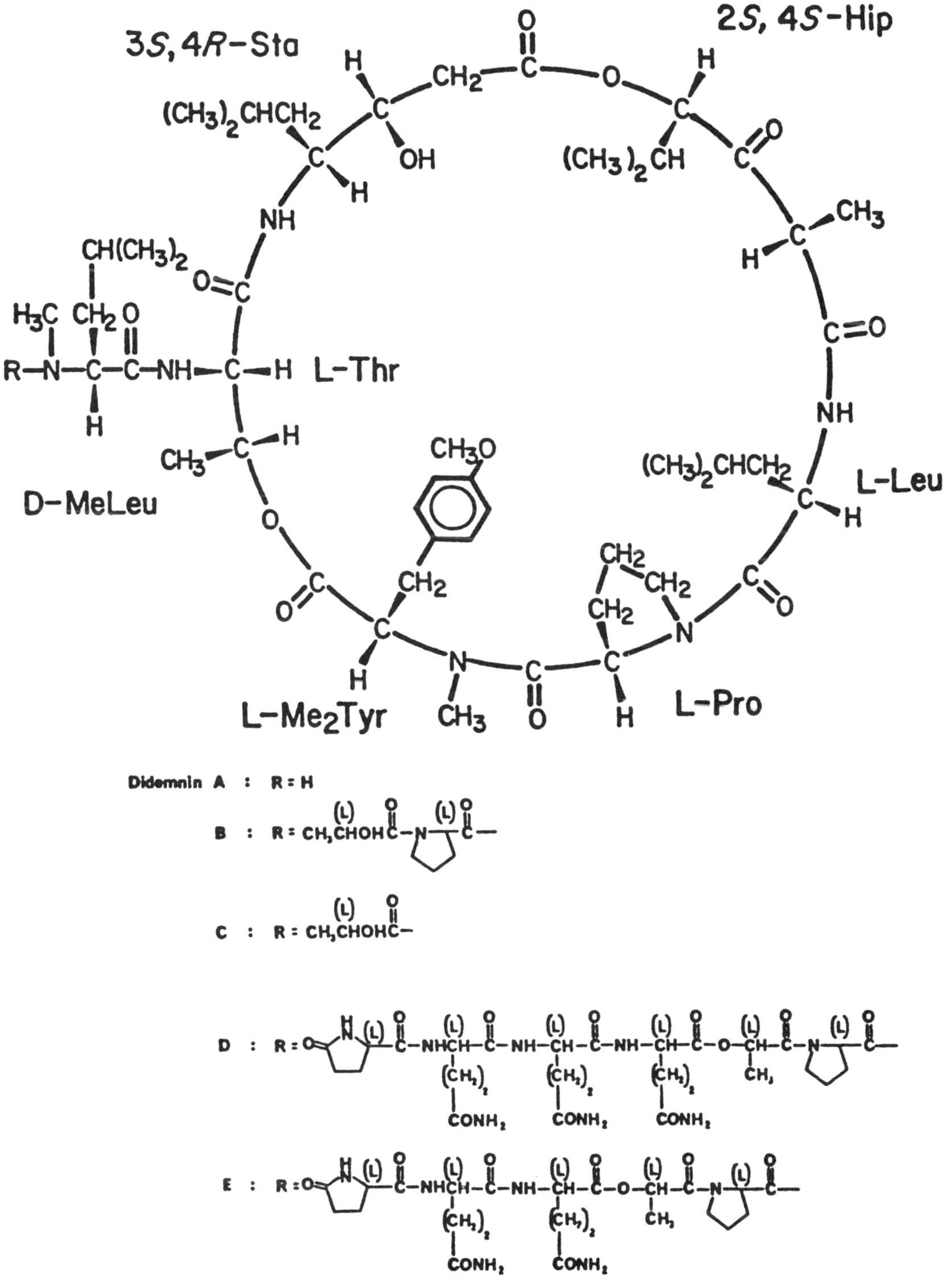

Scheme IV. Structures of the Didemnins.

The isolated natural products became the models for the arabinosides in current clinical use (Ara-C and Ara-A, see structures in Scheme III). A good bit of synthetic chemistry was employed in making analogues of spongothymidine and spongouridine, but as early as 1961 the antitumor properties of Ara-C were well established[48] and in 1977 the *in vivo* antiviral activity of Ara-A against *Herpes* encephalitis was demonstrated.[49] Other aspects of the story have been reviewed by Cohen.[50]

15-*epi*-PGA_2. Another serendipitous discovery occurred during the extensive investigation by Weinheimer and Ciereszko of the terpenes of gorgonians.[51] In 1969, Weinheimer and Spraggins isolated from the gorgonian *Plexaura homomalla* a non-terpenoid metabolite, the prostaglandin 15-*epi*-PGA_2, whose structure is shown below.[52] For a time this discovery stimulated enormous activity, both in looking at gorgonians for prostaglandins and in converting 15-*epi*-PGA_2, present at up to 5% of the weight of the gorgonian, to other prostaglandins.[53] Ultimately, however, totally synthetic procedures proved more fruitful for the preparation of prostaglandins and, except for studies of biosynthesis,[54] this potentially rich source was abandoned. The lesson to be learned here is that total synthesis can provide an effective competition as well as a complementary source for natural products of sufficient interest.

Didemnin B. The cyclic depsipeptide didemnin B (see structure in Scheme IV)[55] is the most active compound isolated from the *Trididemnum* tunicate whose antitumor and antiviral activities were discovered during the 1978 Alpha Helix Caribbean Expedition.[26] During that expedition, the tunicate was shown on site to have both activities, which were reproducible. Didemnin B was subsequently found to be active *in vitro* and *in vivo* against both DNA viruses such as *Herpes simplex* virus, type 2, and RNA viruses such as Rift Valley fever virus. Didemnin B's activity against Rift Valley fever virus is similar to that of ribavirin but at a dose 1000-fold less.[56] Moreover, it was demonstrated to be active both *in vitro* and *in vivo* against L1210 and P388 leukemia and melanoma and is currently in Phase I clinical trials sponsored by the National Cancer Institute.* Didemnin B is also highly immunosuppressive, differing in details but showing in some respects the same activity as cyclosporin A, but at orders of magnitude lower concentrations.[57]

In summary, despite a lack of Western folkloric history of drugs from the sea, there have been successes with marine-derived compounds in the pharmaceutical area, deriving both from extensive bioassay-directed screening programs and from serendipitous discoveries of unusual structural types. The most successful compounds thus far are based on synthetic modification of those unusual structural types.

REFERENCES

1. "Drugs from the Sea", Freudenthal, H.D., Ed., J. Ocean Technol., Marine Technol. Soc., Washington, D.C., 1968.
2. "Food-Drugs from the Sea Proceedings 1969", Youngken, H.W., Jr., Ed., Marine Technol. Soc., Washington, D.C., 1970.
3. "Food-Drugs from the Sea Proceedings 1972", Worthen, L.R., Ed., Marine Technol. Soc., Washington, D.C., 1973.
4. "Food-Drugs from the Sea Proceedings 1974", Webber, H.H. and Ruggieri, G.D., Eds., Marine Technol. Soc., Washington, D.C., 1976.
5. "Drugs & Food from the Sea", Kaul, P.N. and Sindermann, C.J., Eds., The University of Oklahoma Press, Norman, OK, 1978.

* Phase II clinical trials, again sponsored by the NCI, are scheduled to begin in mid-1987.

6. Baslow, M.H., "Marine Pharmacology. A Study of Toxins and Other Biologically Active Substances of Marine Origin", Williams & Wilkins Co., Baltimore, MD, 1969.
7. "Bioactive Compounds from the Sea", Humm, H.J. and Lane, C.E., Eds., Marcel Dekker, Inc., New York, 1974.
8. Hashimoti, Y., "Marine Toxins and Other Bioactive Marine Metabolites", Japan Scientific Societies Press, Tokyo, 1979.
9. Scheuer, P.J., "Chemistry of Marine Natural Products", Academic Press, New York, 1973; "Marine Natural Products. Chemical and Biological Perspectives", Scheuer, P.J., Ed., Academic Press, New York, Vols. I and II, 1978; Vol. II, 1980; Vol. IV, 1981; Vol. V, 1983.
10. Faulkner, D.J., *Nat. Prod. Rep.*, 1984, *1*, 251, 551.
11. "Biomedical Applications of the Horseshoe Crab (Limulidae)", Cohen, E., Ed., A.R. Liss, Inc., New York, 1979.
12. Abraham, E.P., *Pharmacol. Rev.*, 1962, *14*, 473.
13. Kreig, M.D., "Green Medicine", Rand McNally, Chicago, 1964.
14. Morton, J.F., "Major Medicinal Plants", C.C. Thomas, Springfield, IL, 1977.
15. Balandrin, M.F.; Klocke, J.A.; Wurtele, E.S.; Bollinger, W.H., *Science (Washington, D.C.)*, 1985, *228*, 1154.
16. Ruggieri, G.D., *Ibid.*, 1976, *194*, 491.
17. Connor, J.L., Abstracts, Western Society of Naturalists, Monterey, CA, Dec. 27-29, 1985.
18. "Dictionary of Chinese Medicine", Shanghai Scientific Technology Publisher, Shanghai, Vols. I and II, 1977; Supplement, 1979.
19. Halstead, B.W., "Poisonous and Venomenous Marine Animals of the World", U.S. Government Printing Office, Washington, D.C., Vol. I, Invertebrates, 1965; Vol. II, Vertebrates, 1967 and 1970.
20. Fuhrman, F.A., *Sci. Amer.*, 1967, *217*, 60-52, 67.
21. "NOAA Diving Manual. Diving for Science and Technology", U.S. Government Printing Office, Washington, D.C., 1975, p. 10-11.
22. Busby, R.F., "Manned Submersibles", Office of the Oceanographer of the Navy, Washington, D.C., 1976.
23. Rinehart, K.L., Jr.; Armstrong, J.E.; Hughes, R.G., Jr.; Thiess, W.C.; Munro, M.H.G.; Holt, T.G.; Hummel, H.; Pomponi, S.A., Abstracts, IUPAC Fifth International Symposium on Marine Natural Products, Paris, France, September 2-6, 1985.
24. "Alpha Helix Research Program", University of California, San Diego, CA, 1971.
25. Shaw, P.D.; McClure, W.O.; Van Blaricom, G; Sims, J.; Fenical, W.; Rude, J., in Ref. 4, pp 429-433; Rinehart, K.L., Jr.; Johnson, R.D.; Paul, I.C.; McMillan, J.A.; Siuda, J.F.; Krejcarek, G.E., in Ref. 4, pp 434-442.
26. Rinehart, K.L., Jr.; Shaw, P.D.; Shield, L.S.; Gloer, J.B.; Harbour, G.C.; Koker, M.E.S.; Samain, D.; Schwartz, R.E.; Tymiak, A.A.; Weller, D.L.; Carter, G.T.; Munro, M.H.G.; Hughes, R.G., Jr., Renis, E.H.; Swynenberg, E.B.; Stringfellow, D.A.; Vavra, J.J.; Coats, J.H.; Zurenko, G.E.; Kuentzel, S.L.; Li, L.H.; Bakus, G.J.; Brusca, R.C.; Craft, L.L.; Young, D.N.; Connor, J.L., *Pure Appl. Chem.*, 1981, *53*, 795.
27. Shield, L.S.; Rinehart, K.L., Jr., in "Antibiotics: Isolation, Separation and Purification", Weinstein, M.J.; Wagman, G.H., Eds., Elsevier, Amsterdam, 1978, pp 309-385.
28. Higgs, M.D.; Faulkner, D.J., *J. Org. Chem.*, 1978, *43*, 3454.
29. Phillipson, D.W.; Rinehart, K.L., Jr., *J. Am. Chem. Soc.*, 1983, *105*, 7735.
30. Jakowska, S.; Nigrelli, R.F., *N.Y. Acad. Sci.*, 1960, *90*, 913-916.
31. Burkholder, P.R., in Ref. 1, pp 87-112.
32. Faulkner, D.J., in "Topics in Antibiotic Chemistry", Sammes, P.G., Ed., Vol. 2, Ellis Horwood, Ltd., Chichester, U.K., 1978, pp 9-58.

33. Pettit, G.R.; Day, J.F. Hartwell, J.L., Wood, H.B., *Nature (London)*, 1970, *227*, 962.
34. Weinheimer, A.J.; Karns, T.K.B., in Ref. 4, pp 491-496; Weinheimer, A.J.; Matson, J.A.; Karns, T.K.B.; Hossain, M.B.; van der Helm, D., in Ref. 5, pp 117-121.
35. Pettit, G.R., "Biosynthetic Products for Cancer Chemotherapy", Vol. 1, Plenum Press, New York, 1977, Chap. 9 and 10; Pettit, G.R.; Cragg, G.M., "Biosynthetic Products for Cancer Chemotherapy", Vol. 2, Plenum Press, New York, 1978, Chap. 7 and 8; Pettit, G.R.; Ode, R.H., "Biosynthetic Products for Cancer Chemotherapy", Vol. 3, Plenum Press, New York, 1979, Chap. 7 and 8; Pettit, G.R.; Craig, G.M.; Herald, C.L., "Biosynthetic Products for Cancer Chemistry", Elsevier, Amsterdam, Vol. 4, 1984, and Vol. 5, 1985, chap. 2, 9, 10 and 18 in Vol. 4 and 9-11 and 19-21 in Vol. 5.
36. "Antitumor Compounds of Natural Origin: Chemistry and Biochemistry," Vol. 1, Aszalos, A., Ed., CRC Press, Boca Raton, FL, 1981, Chap. 1.
37. Rinehart, K.L., Jr.; Gloer, J.B.; Hugues, R.G., Jr., Renis, H.E.; McGovren, J.P.; Swynenberg, E.B.; Stringfellow, D.A.; Kuentzel, S.L.; Li, L.H., *Science (Washington, D.C.)*, 1981, *212*, 933.
38. Pettit, G.R.; Kamano, Y.; Brown, P.; Gust, D.; Inoue, M.; Herald, C.L., *J. Am. Chem. Soc.*, 1982, *104*, 905.
39. Hamada, Y.; Kohda, K.; Shiori, T., *Tetrahedron Lett.*, 1984, *25*, 5303; Schmidt, U.; Utz, R., *Angew. Chem.*, 1984, *96*, 723.
40. Sigel, M.M.; Wellham, L.L.; Lichter, W.; Dudeck, L.E.; Gargus, J.L.; Lucas, A.H., in Ref. 2, pp 281-29; Sigel, M.M.; McCumber, L.J.; Hightower, J.A.; Hayasaka, S.S.; Huggins, E.M., Jr.; Davis, J.F., *Amer. Zool.*, 1983, *23*, 221 and references therein.
41. Holt, T.G.; Rinehart, K.L., Jr., unpublished results.
42. Rinehart, K.L., Jr.; Kobayashi, J.; Harbour, G.C.; Hugues, R.G., Jr.; Miszak, S.A.; Scahill, T.A., *J. Am. Chem. Soc.*, 1984, *106*, 1524; Kobayashi, J.; Harbour, G.C.; Gilmore, J.; Rinehart, K.L., Jr., *J. Am. Chem. Soc.*, 1984, *106*, 1526.
43. Kaul, P.N.; Kulkarni, S.K.; Schmitz, F.J.; Hollenbeak, K.H., in Ref. 5, pp 99-106.
44. Shibata, S.; Dunn, D.F.; Kuchii, M.; Kashiwagi, M.; Norton, T.R., *J. Pharm. Sci.*, 1974, *63*, 1332; Norton, T.R.; Kashiwagi, M.; Shibata, S., in Ref. 5, pp 37-50 and references therein.
45. Beress, L., in Ref. 5, pp 59-72 and references therein.
46. Endo, M., in Ref. 23
47. Bergmann, W.; Feeney, R.J., *J. Am. Chem. Soc.*, 1950, *72*, 2809; Bergmann, W.; Feeney, R.J., *J. Org. Chem.*, 1951, *16*, 981.
48. Evans, J.S.; Musser, E.A.; Mengel, G.D.; Forsblad, K.R.; Hunter, J.H., *Proc. Soc. Exptl. Biol. Med.*, 1961, *106*, 350.
49. Whitley, R.J.; Soong, S.-J.; Dolin, R.; Galasso, G.J.; Ch'ien, L.T.; Alford, C.A.; Collaborative Study Group. *New England J. Med.*, 1977, *297*, 289.
50. Cohen, S.S., in "Progress in Nucleic Acid Research and Molecular Biology", Davidson, J.N.; Cohn, W.D., Eds, Academic Press, New York, 1966, Vol. 5, pp 1-88, and references therein.
51. Ciereszko, L.S.; Karns, T.K.B., in "Biology and Geology of Coral Reefs", Vol. II: Biology 1, Jones, O.A.; Endean, R., Eds., Academic Press, New York, 1973, pp 183-203; Tursch, B.; Braekman, J.C.; Daloze, D.; Kaisin, M., in Ref. 9, Vol. II, pp 247-296.
52. Weinheimer, A.J.; Spraggins, R.L., *Tetrahedron Lett.* 1969, 5185.
53. Crabbé, P., *Chem. Britain*, 1975, *11*, 132; Nelson, N.A.; Kelly, R.C.; Johnson, R.A., *Chem. Eng. News*, 1982, August 16, pp 30-44.
54. Corey, E.J.; Shimoji, K.; Shih, C., *J. Am. Chem. Soc.*, 1984, *106*, 6425.

55. Canonico, P.G.; Pannier, W.L.; Huggins, J.W.; Rinehart, K.L., Jr., *Antimicrob. Agents Chemother.*, 1982, *22*, 696.
56. Rinehart, K.L., Jr.; Gloer, J.B.; Wilson, G.R.; Hughes, R.G., Jr.; Li, L.H.; Renis, H.E.; McGovren, J.P., *Fed. Proc.*, 1983, *42*, 87.
57. Montgomery, D.W.; Zukowski, C.F., *Transplantation*, 1985, *40*, 49.

Alexander Leaf
Department of Preventive Medicine, Harvard Medical School, Massachusetts General Hospital, Boston, Massachusetts 02114, U.S.A.

Fish Oil and Human Nutrition

The role of fish and fish oils in the prevention of atherosclerosis and particularly in the prevention of heart attack is of great medical and popular interest. In order to set this interest in proper perspective I would like to describe briefly the burden of illness represented by coronary artery disease.

Coronary artery disease (CAD) is the major cause of death and morbidity in the United States and in most Western industrialized countries. According to the most recent figures,[1] 4.7 million Americans have coronary artery disease, either a past myocardial infarction or angina pectoris. It is predicted that *ca.* 1.5 million Americans will suffer a heart attack this year and about 550,000 will die. Furthermore, nearly 350,000 victims will die before reaching a hospital. Thus, despite a very gratifying 25% reduction in mortality rate from CAD in the United States since 1967, CAD remains the leading cause of death and a major cause of morbidity in the United States. According to estimates of the American Heart Association, the total cost of medical care for cardiovascular diseases in the United States, including hospitalization, physicians' charges, medications, and lost output due to disability, will be $72.1 billion in 1985. Coronary artery disease accounts for a large portion of these costs, and other industrialized, developed countries suffer a similar burden of illness, some even greater than ours. Furthermore, the reduction in mortality rate that has occurred in the United States in the past 20 years has not occurred in all afflicted countries. Some have continued to experience increasing coronary artery disease mortality rates.

Against this burden of illness, the 1972 report by Danish physicians Bang and Dyerberg[2] of their epidemiologic and plasma lipid studies among the Eskimos of Greenland was noteworthy. They found the age-adjusted mortality rate from heart attacks among the Greenland Eskimos to be approximately 1/8 the corresponding rates in Denmark and the United States, that is, 5.3% of all deaths *vs.* 40.4% in the United States and 34.7% in Denmark during 1974-76.[3] Such a low incidence of coronary artery disease would not be unusual for many parts of the underdeveloped world, but the Eskimo diet has a very high content of seal, walrus, and whale meat, as well as some fish, and is very high in protein and fat. A high incidence of atherosclerosis and heart attack would be expected in a population consuming such a highly atherogenic diet. In fact, some 40% of the calories taken in by the Greenland Eskimos and the Danes are derived from fats;[3] this is comparable to the average American diet.

Analyses of the composition of dietary fat, however, revealed striking differences between the Eskimo and Danish diets. First, the Danes consumed about twice as much saturated fat as did the Eskimos--53% *vs.* 23% of total fatty acids.[3] Second, the consumption of N - 6 and N - 3 fatty acids differed in the two populations, an important finding, which we will discuss here. The Danes consumed more N - 6 and less N - 3 polyunsaturated fatty acid than did the Eskimos.

Since the incidence of coronary artery disease in the Western developed nations is directly proportional to the amount of saturated fat and cholesterol in the diet, Dyerberg looked to the cholesterol levels in the two populations and indeed found that at all ages Eskimo men and women had a lower total cholesterol level than did the Danes.[2] However, the lower cholesterol level among the Eskimos was not sufficient to account for the markedly lower incidences of coronary artery disease deaths in that population. Thus, the basis for the lower mortality from heart attacks was sought elsewhere, and the current explanation seems to involve the particular role of marine oils, namely the N - 3 fatty acids.

There are three main dietary classes of polyunsaturated fatty acids. The N - 3 fatty acids are derived from marine sources where N - 3 indicates that the first double bond occurs at the third carbon from the methyl end of the fatty acid; the older nomenclature was ω-3. They are originally synthesized by phytoplankton, enter the food chain through fish, and are high in content in the fat deposits of marine animals who live on fish. Representative important fatty acids of marine origin include eicosapentaenoic acid (EPA, C20:5 N - 3) and docosahexaenoic acid (DHA, C22:6 N - 3). The N - 6 fatty acids are derived largely from vegetable sources. In corn oil, safflower oil, and soy bean oil, for example, the polyunsaturated fatty acids are largely of the N - 6 series. The N - 9 fatty acids, of lesser nutritional significance, occur in vegetables and some animals.

The significance of the N - 3 fatty acids in relation to the low incidence of coronary artery disease seems to be their effect upon prostaglandin metabolism. Prostaglandins are chemical messengers which are synthesized within most cells of the body. They are not stored in the cells but are synthesized in response to a variety of hormonal and other stimuli and are released into the extracellular fluid where they mediate their potent effects upon neighboring cells. Their half-life in their active form is so brief that they do not exist in this form in significant concentrations within the circulating blood. In response to a variety of stimuli, including hormonal stimuli, arachidonic acid is released enzymatically by phospholipases from phospholipids. In the endothelium of arteries the released arachidonic acid is metabolized *via* the cyclooxygenase pathway to produce prostacyclin (PGI_2), a potent vasodilator, PGI_2 is antiaggregatory for platelets, thus preventing the formation of blood clots. However, in platelets, small non-nucleated cells which circulate in the blood and initiate blood clotting, the arachidonic acid is metabolized *via* cyclooxygenase to form thromboxane (TXA_2). Thromboxane is one of the most potent vasodilators known, and it also aggregates platelets. Thus, the balance of formation on the one hand of prostacyclin, which is antiaggregatory, and on the other hand of thromboxane, which aggregates platelets, is important to coagulation.

When animals are fed a diet containing the N - 3 fatty acids, eicosapentaenoic acid displaces arachidonic acid in the phospholipids of cell and platelet plasma membranes.[4] Furthermore, this eicosapentaenoic acid, which is released by phospholipases along with arachidonic acid from phospholipids, competes with arachidonic acid. In the endothelial cells lining the arteries, EPA does not reduce but enhances the formation of prostacyclins.[5] In platelets, however, EPA inhibits the formation of thromboxane from arachidonic acid to give small amounts of EPA-generated thromboxane[6] which appears to be physiologically inactive. This competition of EPA with arachidonic acid disrupts the usual balance between prostacyclin and thromboxane. The result is an increase in the amount of thromboxane, which is proaggregatory--aggregation of platelets is thereby inhibited.

The prevention of platelet aggregation is important to atherogenesis.[7] The initial event in the formation of atherosclerosis is injury to arterial endothelium. In the absence of endothelial cells, platelets exposed to underlying collagen release thromboxane and aggregate at the site of the endothelial injury where they release a platelet-derived growth factor (PDGF). This growth factor stimulates the multiplication of the underlying smooth muscle cells in the media and their migration to the site of the injury. It also causes monocytes/macrophages to migrate to the site of the injury and to multiply there. In the presence of excess plasma cholesterol, cholesterol is deposited within the smooth muscle cells and the macrophages produce foam cells which, together with an increase in interstitial connective tissue and thrombus formation, gradually accrete and cause narrowing of the arterial lumen with atheromatous lesions. Repetition of endothelial injury, with platelet aggregation and formation of foam cells and thrombi, gradually narrows and eventually occludes the blood vessels. In the heart, this results in coronary artery disease, myocardial infarction, and, all too often, death. A bruising tendency, but no clinically manifest bleeding,[8] has been noted among Greenland Eskimos; their prolonged bleeding time is an indication of the reduced aggregability of their platelets.

Several clinical studies in humans support this postulated action of eicosapentaenoic acid on prostacyclin and thromboxane production.[4-6,9] Normal humans fed either a high fish diet or a diet supplemented with fish oil also develop prolonged bleeding times; prostacyclin production by their blood vessels is increased, but thromboxane production is markedly inhibited. The change in platelet aggregation in response to adenosine diphosphate, collagen, or catecholamines, three agents which normally effect rapid platelet aggregation, is much less in individuals ingesting fish or fish oils.

Since the initial step in the development of atherosclerosis involves aggregation of platelets at a site of endothelial injury,[7] the failure of platelets to aggregate can prevent atherosclerosis. This is now thought to be the main means by which fish and fish oils protect the Greenland Eskimos from atherosclerosis, despite the high levels of fat in their diet.

Since most fatty acids in oils of marine origin are polyunsaturated, it would be expected that plasma levels of total and LDL cholesterol would also be reduced on ingestion of fish oils. The plasma cholesterol levels of the Eskimos were, in fact, significantly lower than those of the Danes. Thus far, in clinical studies of relatively short duration (3-12 weeks) using low doses of N - 3 fatty acids, variable effects upon the plasma cholesterol levels have been observed. However, in patients with combined hyperlipidemia due to elevated levels of both triglycerides and cholesterol (Types IIB and V hyperlipidemias, respectively) the administration of fish oils such as salmon to yield 20-30 grams per day of N - 3 fatty acid produced a marked reduction in both triglycerides and LDL cholesterol levels.[10] A 20-year study in Holland[11] of 852 males free of clinical coronary artery disease at the initiation of the study in 1960 revealed an inverse relationship between the mortality rate from heart attacks and the amount of fish ingested, over a range from 0 to more than 45 grams of fish per day. The age-adjusted incidence of coronary heart disease among those ingesting the larger amounts of fish was approximately 1/3 that among individuals who ate no fish. The effect of fish consumption on mortality from coronary heart disease remains statistically significant after the data were corrected for other cardiovascular risk factors known to be operable among the males studied. It was concluded that ingesting one or two fish meals per week could significantly reduce the risk of death from coronary artery disease. The amount of N - 3 fatty acid ingested by males, who were partially protected from coronary artery disease mortality, after consuming relatively small average amounts of fish seems too small to confer such protection; this raises the question of the role of other ingredients in fish in preventing coronary atherosclerosis.

At this time there is good epidemiologic evidence that N - 3 fatty acids derived from marine sources can produce significant protection against heart attacks. There are, however, many aspects of this role of the fatty acids which need further investigation. We do not yet know how much N - 3 fatty acids are required to protect an individual from a heart attack. We do not know whether a supplement of N - 3 fatty acids can be simply added to the Western diet nor whether the N - 3 fatty acids will only be protective if there is a sharp simultaneous reduction in the quantity of N - 6 fatty acids ingested. Data to date suggest at least that the effect of N - 3 fatty acids in preventing atherosclerosis is increased by a concomitant reduction in N - 6 fatty acids and, of course, in saturated fatty acids. We do not yet have the answers to many other questions, but at least the direction of research is visible.

I have devoted a major portion of my presentation to consideration of the favorable effects of N - 3 fatty acids from marine sources upon the prevention of the major cause of death and morbidity in the United States and Western industrialized countries, but the story goes beyond coronary artery disease. Arachidonic acid, the usual N - 6 fatty acid, is metabolized not only by the cyclooxygenase pathway, but also by the lipoxygenase enzymatic pathway to give the leukotrienes, chemical messengers which are potent in modulating the inflammatory response. When eicosapentaenoic acid replaces arachidonic acid in plasma membranes, the eicosapentaenoic acid is also metabolized by the lipoxygenase pathway to give marked changes in leukotriene production[12] and significant modulation of some inflammatory and immune responses. It has been shown, for example, that autoimmune disease can be almost completely prevented in a strain of mice with a genetic tendency to an autoimmune renal disease and early death from uremia by changing the fat in their diet from the usual animal sources to fish oils.[13] Clinical studies are under way to assess the effect of fish oil feeding upon human autoimmune diseases, including lupus erythematosus, asthma, and other inflammatory diseases such as rheumatoid arthritis and psoriasis; even experimental cancer can be modified by fish oil feedings. It is exciting to know that simple dietary measures can so profoundly influence the major diseases.

REFERENCES

1. American Heart Association. Heart Facts, 1985, pp 1-25.
2. Bang, H.O.; Dyerberg, J., *Acta Med. Scand.*, 1972, *192*, 85.
3. Dyerberg, J., in *Nutritional Evaluations of Long-Chain Fatty Acids in Fish Oil*, Barlow, S.M.; Stansby, M.E., Eds., Academic Press, 1982, pp 245-261.
4. Goodnight, S.H.; Harris, W.S.; Connor, W.E.; Illingworth, D.R., *Arteriosclerosis*, 1982, *2*, 87.
5. Fischer, S.; Weber, P.C., *Nature (London)*, 1984, *307*, 165.
6. Fischer, S.; Weber, P.C., *Biochem. Biophys. Res. Commun.*, 1983, *116*, 1091.
7. Ross, R.; Faggiotto, A.; Bowen-Pope, D.; *et al., Circulation*, 1984, *70* (suppl.), *77*.
8. Dyerberg, J.; Bang, H.O., *Lancet*, 1979, *2*, 433.
9. Goodnight, S.H.; Harris, W.S.; Connor, W.E., *Blood*, 1981, *58*, 880.
10. Phillipson, B.E.; Rothrock, D.W.; Connor, W.E.; *et al., New Engl. J. Med*, 1985, *82*, 1210.
11. Kromhout, D.; Bosschieter, E.B.; Goulander, C.de L., *New Engl. J. Med.*, 1985, *312*, 1205.
12. Lee, T.H.; Hoover, R.L.; Williams, J.D.; *et al., New Engl. J. Med.*, 1985, *312*, 1217.
13. Pricket, J.D.; Robinson, D.R.; Steinberg, A.D., *J. Clin. Invest.*, 1981, *68*, 566.

Section II

Needs and Prospects for New Pharmaceutical Agents from Marine Sources

Irving P. Delappe
Molecular Microbiology and Parasitology Branch, National Institute of Allergy and Infectious Diseases, National Institutes of Health, Bethesda, Maryland 20892, U.S.A.

New Agents Needed for Infectious Diseases

During the past 30 years, the health problems created by bacterial resistance to antibiotics have become strikingly apparent. Hospital-associated or nosocomial infections attributable to *Staphylococcus* organism are increasingly difficult to control, and sexually transmitted diseases, one of which is caused by *Gonococcus* bacterium, represent another important problem. Both of these infections would be far more widespread were it not for basic research, supported by the National Institute of Allergy and Infectious Diseases (one of the National Institutes of Health in Bethesda, Maryland), on the mechanisms of resistance to antimicrobial agents and on the isolation of new antibiotics from natural products followed by determination of their structure with the ultimate goal of synthesis.

The Molecular Microbiology and Parasitology Branch of the National Institute of Allergy and Infectious Diseases administers approximately 500 research support mechanisms, amounting to about $56,000,000 in 1985, including grants, training grants, career development awards, fellowships, and contracts in the above scientific areas, almost all of which involve basic science. This money is divided approximately equally between the two sections of the Branch, Molecular Microbiology and Parasitology.

MOLECULAR MICROBIOLOGY

Activities in this section may be placed in three categories:

(a) Mechanisms of resistance to antimicrobial agents. The principal goal of this program is to elucidate fundamental biological mechanisms involved in the development of drug resistance in microorganisms and to increase our basic understanding of this phenomenon. Specific goals of this program involve investigation of the origin, development, evolution, expression, and mechanism of drug resistance in a variety of specific microorganisms. Bacterial plasmids occupy a dominant role in the study of resistance.

(b) Recombinant DNA molecules (genetic engineering). The primary goal of this program is the development and utilization of recombinant DNA molecule technology to increase fundamental knowledge and ultimately enhance our control of the etiological agents of infectious diseases. Another goal is the synthesis of a variety of biologically useful substances through the construction of bacterial cells containing functional DNA of either plant or animal origin. Equally important goals are the identification, assessment, and elimination of all biohazards encountered in the exploitation of this technology.

(c) Isolation of novel and promising antibiotics from natural products and ultimate synthesis based on structure determination. For the purpose of this meeting the third category is of paramount importance, but it must be remembered that the increased activity in this area has been the result, to a great extent, of the need to deal with widespread resistance to antimicrobial agents.

PARASITOLOGY

This section of the Branch has research interests in the areas of parasitology, medical entomology (insect vectors of parasites, for the most part), and tropical diseases (exotic diseases not normally found within the borders of the United States).

Activities in this section can be placed in two categories:

(a) Immunology of parasitic infections. Major goals of studies on immunology of parasitic infections are the development of effective vaccines for the prevention of parasitic diseases (*e.g.*, malaria, schistosomiasis, and filariasis); the intervention of the host response to prevent or ameliorate disease processes which are immunologically mediated; and the development or improvement of immunodiagnostic procedures for parasitic infections, especially relating to the immune status of the host.

(b) Biological regulation of vectors. This program has as its goal the advancement of fundamental studies which might lead to effective methods for the biological control of vectors.

One may wonder why the parasitology section of the Branch is relevant to this meeting; there is a valid rationale for this. *Giardia lambia*, a pathogen of increasing importance in recent years, is the causative agent for giardiasis, an intestinal disease whose pathogenesis varies among individuals and has not been adequately explained. Little is known about the immunological events occurring in the intestine and the immune status of the host in terms of disease severity. There is a definite need for stimulation of research on this disease, which is widespread in the United States and in travelers returning from abroad. The drug of choice for treatment of giardiasis is quinacrine hydrochloride (atabrine); alternatives are metronidazole and furazolidone. Metronidazole is carcinogenic in rodents and mutagenic in bacteria and should not be given to pregnant women, especially in the first trimester. A better understanding of the immunology of giardiasis would allow more efficient diagnosis, assessment of treatment, and characterization of strains of the parasite in relation to pathogenicity.

Amebiasis, while not as common as giardiasis, is still present in this country. Little is known about differences in strains of amebae as they relate to invasiveness and pathogenicity. Characteristics such as increased erythrophagocytosis, surface binding, and surface charge have been identified in potentially pathogenic strains, but further study is necessary to understand better the conditions that modulate disease production. Expansion of studies of *Entamoeba histolytica* isolates would help achieve this goal. Better identification of virulent strains of *E. histolytica* would aid in detection and management of the disease and would be of value in epidemiological studies.

The drug of choice in treating early asymptomatic amebiasis is iodoquinol. Maximum dosage of iodoquinol should not exceed two grams per day, and treatment should not be prolonged because of the possibility of optic neuritis. Treatments for mild to moderate intestinal disease, severe intestinal disease, or hepatic abscess are described in *The Medical Letter on Drugs and Therapeutics*, 1984, *26*.

In another instance, acquired immune deficiency syndrome (AIDS) is currently the most feared communicable disease in this country. The Center for Disease Control (CDC) in Atlanta, Georgia, estimated in a July 26, 1985, report that there were 12,067 cases, with

6,079 deaths to date. In a very large number of cases, once AIDS is present and the immune defenses are lowered measurably, two usually innocuous protozoan parasites, *Pneumocystis carinii* and *Cryptosporidium* sp., take advantage of the body's lowered defenses and complicate an already bad situation. Both are opportunistic parasites; *Pneumocystis carinii* in the lung is a prime cause of death in AIDS patients, whereas *Cryptosporidium* brings about an intractable diarrhea. In the case of *P. carinii*, trimethoprim (structurally related to pyrimethamine) has been used in various combinations with sulfamethoxazole with varying degrees of success. Pentamidine is an effective, but highly toxic, chemotherapeutic agent. AIDS patients with pneumocystis pneumonia have not responded well to either treatment. *Cryptosporidium* infections, thus far, have not been responsive to drugs.

Of interest to the Molecular Microbiology section of the Branch are the allergenic properties of the beta-lactams, penicillins and cephalosporins; from personal experience I know that the latter can cause a bad rash, alleviated only by use of an antihistamine, benadryl. Representatives of this group are now used widely for prophylaxis after surgery where there is the possibility of nosocomial infections (*e.g.*, *Staphylococcus aureus*). Non-allergenic antibiotics are badly needed in this area; perhaps new natural products from the sea could help solve this problem.

Cystic fibrosis is an inherited recessive trait with a one in four chance of developing in infants of either sex if both parents are carriers. Its etiology is unknown. The average incidence is about 1 in 1500 and it strikes Caucasian children predominantly. It features abnormally viscid mucus secretions in its respiratory stage, and eventually the larger bronchi are filled with purulent secretions. Although *S. aureus* has been incriminated in a large number of cases, evidence for *Pseudomonas aeruginosa* involvement is growing.

The National Institute of Allergy and Infectious Diseases, through a contract support mechanism, hopes to initiate a series of clinical trials involving antibiotic prophylaxis in infants with cystic fibrosis. These trials will involve a comparison of cephalexin, a cephalosporin, with a placebo to prevent bacterial (*P. aeruginosa*) colonization and subsequent pulmonary dysfunction in newly diagnosed infants. Cephalexin is useful, when oral therapy is feasible, for certain infections of the respiratory tract. This clinical trial is necessary to evaluate the effect of continuous cephalexin prophylaxis on morbidity, pulmonary function, and physical growth of cystic fibrosis patients. Such use is not without risk however, since anaphylaxis has followed the administration of cephalosporins to penicillin-sensitive patients.

An estimated 800 million chronic hepatitis B carriers worldwide could be aided by the development of antiviral compounds. Basic research has identified potential steps of viral replication that could be inhibited by specific drugs. The benefits could include moderation of symptoms, reduction of transmission, diminished progression to more severe sequelae, and decreased health care costs.

Severe cytomegalovirus infection has been particularly unresponsive to most antivirals, including interferon, and it is increasing as the numbers of transplants and AIDS patients rise. Promising drugs are becoming available, but more would be welcome. One is an acyclic nucleoside, 9-(1,3-dihydroxy-2-propoxymethyl)guanine (DHPG) which is synergistic when used in conjunction with recombinant mouse gamma interferon against *Herpes simplex* virus, type 2, in mice.

The incidence of systemic mycotic diseases, such as candidiasis and aspergillosis, continues to rise, especially in immunocompromised patients with other disabling diseases (cancer, AIDS, severe burn and trauma cases, etc.). To combat the heavy burden of morbidity and mortality attributable to these diseases, improved treatments with existing and new antifungal agents must be developed and evaluated scientifically in controlled clinical trials. A clinical trial comparing the imidazole antifungals, ketoconazole and itraconazole, with standard amphotericin B treatment for systemic candidiasis and/or aspergillosis is required. New agents from the sea might help.

Variations in the ability of aminocyclitol antibiotics such as gentamicin to penetrate different bacterial membranes can account for the pharmacologic and toxic profiles of these antibiotics. Gentamicin is the preferred antibiotic for the treatment of gram-negative infections. Its therapeutic usefulness is restricted by kidney toxicity and damage to the 8th cranial nerve (auditory). The antibiotic accumulates in the kidney cortex up to a concentration eighty times greater than that found in the plasma. This leads to extensive tubular necrosis and kidney failure. It is a potent inhibitor of glucose transport, but has no influence on amino acids. Continued analysis of these findings may lead to improved chemotherapeutic procedures involving use of this important antibiotic. Here, once more, a new antibiotic is needed.

Staphylococcus aureus is a serious pathogen whose methicillin-resistant strains are encountered increasingly in U.S. hospitals. Methicillin is a peptide antibiotic related to penicillin. Investigation of methicillin resistance should be supported not only because of its intrinsic scientific interest, but also because of the potential application to clinical medicine. Research involving the molecular basis of methicillin resistance in certain strains of this organism is under way. Molecular genetic analysis of methicillin resistance will be pursued based on a working hypothesis that this phenomenon is caused not by inactivation of the antibiotic by *S. aureus*, but rather by innate or intrinsic alterations in penicillin-binding proteins (PBP), resulting in a low affinity for this type of antibiotic. A new antibiotic from the sea might thwart these arcane alterations.

In the United States, gonorrhea continues to be one of the most commonly reported communicable diseases, with approximately 900,000 cases in 1984. Both men and women can develop disseminated gonococcal infections, the most common form of which is a type of arthritis. It is also a significant factor in pelvic inflammatory disease in women. For many years, penicillin had been an effective treatment for gonorrhea, but some *Gonococcus* strains have become penicillin-resistant. Hence, there is a great need for the development of an effective gonococcal vaccine or new antibiotic.

NIAID now supports 43 research projects involving the isolation of novel and promising antibiotics from natural products. After structure determination, larger amounts can be obtained by synthesis. In recent years, several natural products have been obtained from the floor of the Caribbean Sea and elsewhere in the world (Australia, Florida, Guam, Mexico, New Zealand, Palau, and Ponape). From the Caribbean, one grantee obtains products from certain tunicates (sea squirts, ascidians) and, from elsewhere in the world, a second grantee obtains material from marine sponges and nudibranch molluscs (molluscs without shells or true gills in the adult state). Only natural products obtained from the Caribbean will be discussed here.

From tunicates, natural products termed didemnins have been isolated and their structures determined. Synthetic efforts are under way. Some of these should prove to be valuable antiviral and antitumor agents. One is of particular interest because of its possible use as a new immunosuppressive agent. It has been found to be one thousand times more active than cyclosporin A, currently used for this purpose.

Only three of our 43 grantees are engaged in this promising and intriguing research and attempts should be made to entice at least three additional grantees to divert their attention to natural products derived from marine organisms. If this does not succeed, then additional money might be more attractive. This could be in the form of a "Pharmaceuticals from the Sea" grant program, first year funds for which could be $400,000, the optimal amount, and perhaps $200,000 minimally.

Michael R. Boyd, Robert H. Shoemaker, Gordon M. Cragg, Matthew Suffness
Division of Cancer Treatment, National Cancer Institute, Developmental Therapeutics Program,
Bethesda, Maryland 20892, U.S.A.

New Avenues of Investigation of Marine Biologicals in the Anticancer Drug Discovery Program of the National Cancer Institute

INTRODUCTION

The preclinical drug discovery and development program of the National Cancer Institute (NCI). The primary mission of the NCI's Developmental Therapeutics Program (DTP) is the discovery and preclinical development of promising new anticancer drug candidates. The DTP is centered at the NIH campus at Bethesda, Maryland, and comprises five intramural basic research laboratories (Biological Chemistry, Medicinal Chemistry, Molecular Pharmacology, Biochemical Pharmacology, and Tumor Cell Biology) and eight extramural branches. The extramural branches serve as the focal points for the administration of a comprehensive, contract-supported drug screening and development effort (Fig. 1). The DTP also administers a substantial portfolio of investigator-initiated projects in preclinical drug research, supported through grants and cooperative agreements.

Strategies for anticancer drug discovery: "Rational" drug design *versus* screening. Increasing knowledge of cancer biology continues to provide the basis for many exciting new avenues for research aimed at "rational" drug design. The further elucidation of potential cellular and molecular targets and the exploitation of these targets in the design, synthesis, and/or modification of promising new anticancer agents are central goals of the DTP-sponsored grants and cooperative agreements. Large-scale screening is the NCI's other primary approach to the identification of new compounds with activities against various tumor model systems. Materials come to the screening program from diverse sources, including industry, academe, and individual scientists. Promising leads, identified initially through screening, frequently require optimization through the "rational" approach (*e.g.*, synthetic modifications to improve activity, solubility, pharmacokinetics). Thus, there is most often an essential and intimate interplay between the "rational" and the screening strategies.

Efforts directed toward the discovery and development of new anticancer drugs from natural products are supported both through investigator-initiated mechanisms (*e.g*, grants), as well as through directed, NCI-initiated projects (contracts). However, the large-scale acquisition and screening projects are primarily contract-supported, and, particularly in the case of natural products, the initial detection of a promising bioactive material relies primarily upon screening. Only through the screening process can new or unanticipated kinds of bioactive materials be discovered; these may then be investigated

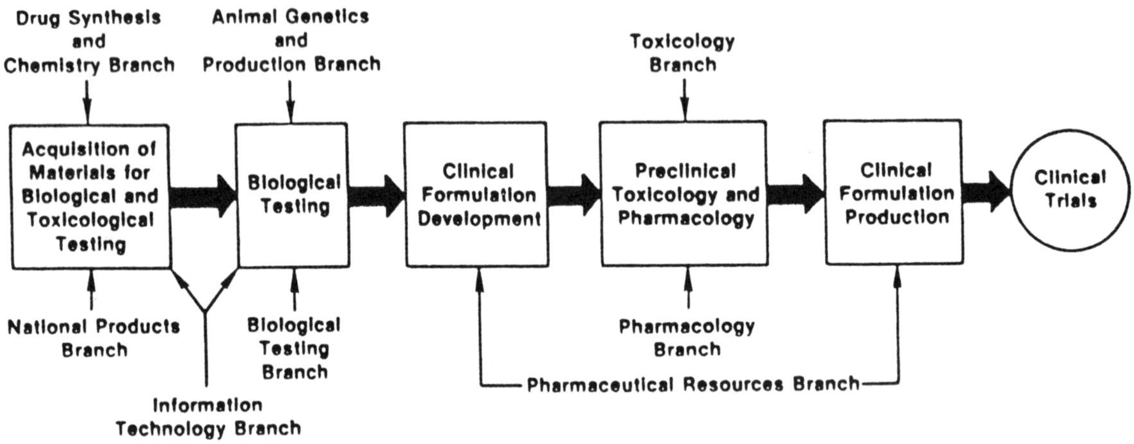
Drug Synthesis and Chemistry Branch
Animal Genetics and Production Branch
Toxicology Branch
Acquisition of Materials for Biological and Toxicological Testing
Biological Testing
Clinical Formulation Development
Preclinical Toxicology and Pharmacology
Clinical Formulation Production
Clinical Trials
National Products Branch
Biological Testing Branch
Pharmacology Branch
Pharmaceutical Resources Branch
Information Technology Branch

Figure 1

further and developed through "rational" approaches. The following discussion focuses, therefore, upon past, present, and future NCI screening programs applicable to natural products. Also specifically addressed are the projected directions for these programs, which will have a major impact on investigations of marine biologicals.

THE NCI "COMPOUND-ORIENTED" DRUG SCREENING PROGRAM 1975-1985

The concept and the approach. The NCI screening program during the period 1975-1985 was an extension of earlier programs based on the view that cytotoxic agents, which destroy rapidly growing tumor cells, may be clinically efficacious against human cancers. Laboratory testing in the 1960's and early 1970's established that a high level of activity in the mouse L1210 leukemia test could be used with moderate success to predict clinical activity *vs.* certain human cancers. Nearly 60% of new compounds brought to clinical trials on this basis later showed positive activity in patients.[1,2] However, the clinical successes were predominantly in treating leukemia, lymphoma, and a very few rare, extremely rapidly growing solid tumors, such as choriocarcinoma, Ewing's sarcoma, and rhabdomyosarcoma.[3] The minimal clinical efficacy or, for most drugs, the total lack of clinical efficacy against slower-growing solid tumors, was a very serious concern, which eventually warranted the adoption of a new strategy. An alternative strategy (Fig. 2) was to screen against a battery of murine tumor models, with particular emphasis on solid tumors, and for the first time, by means of xenografts in athymic mice, on a parallel panel of solid tumors of human origin. As an initial phase of development of the murine tumor panel, available tumor systems were analyzed in detail and the most promising ones were further refined and adapted for mass screening. In particular, the development of the human tumor xenograft systems offered an intriguing new approach to antitumor drug testing.

The screening models 1975-1985. Because of the high cost of *in vivo* testing (particularly in the xenografts) and the large number of models in the tumor panel, it was not possible to screen directly the 10,000 new substances submitted annually. A filter or prescreen was needed to reduce by 90-95% the number of compounds screened in the tumor panel (Fig. 2). The murine P388 lymphocytic leukemia assay selected as an *in vivo* prescreen is highly sensitive to nearly all compounds known to be clinically useful (except steroids and bleomycin) and is more sensitive than the L1210 leukemia assay. Tumor inoculation sites can also be changed relatively easily in order to challenge further those materials showing initial activity. The consensus after considerable testing was that the P388 model was not likely to be overly discriminatory. The prescreen had to be very sensitive, aimed not necessarily at selecting compounds for development but at separating bioactive from biologically inert materials. As the system subsequently operated, approximately 10,000 samples per year were prescreened in the P388 leukemia system, resulting in the identification of about 500 active compounds per year; about 200 of these entered the tumor panel, a reasonable number since many of the initial group were analogues either of known active agents or of each other.

Two steps were taken to minimize any bias arising from the use of a single model (*i.e.*, P388 leukemia) as a prescreen. First, the cutoff criterion for activity in the P388 prescreen was defined as a 20% increase in life span (ILS) in order not to miss any compound with reasonable activity. Second, a "bypass" procedure was established so that compounds which had any known or suspected antiproliferative activity or biochemical mechanism or other biological activity which suggested that they might have anticancer activity were entered into the tumor panel regardless of their performance in the P388 leukemia prescreen.

The screening models utilized at various times for the tumor panel are summarized in Tables 1 and 2. Table 2 shows two levels of activity, the lower of which, MC1, was not

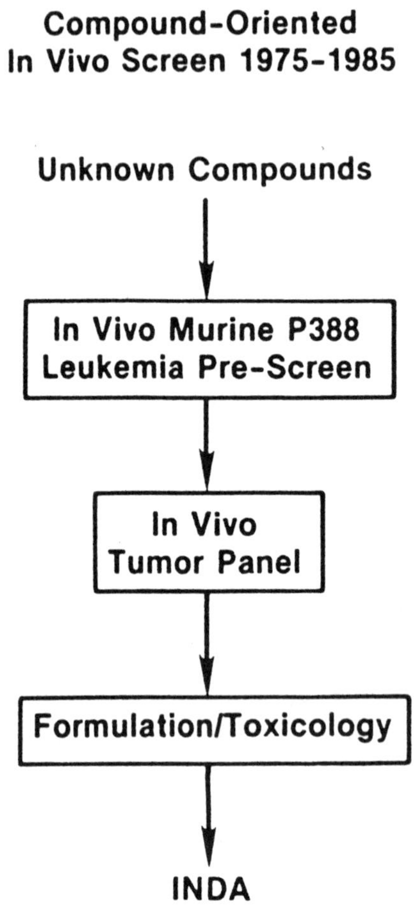
Compound-Oriented
In Vivo Screen 1975-1985
Unknown Compounds
In Vivo Murine P388
Leukemia Pre-Screen
In Vivo
Tumor Panel
Formulation/Toxicology
INDA

Figure 2

Table 1

DCT Prescreen and Tumor Panel Models

Tumor	Test Host	Inoculum	Site
Mouse tumors			
B16 melanoma	BDF_1, $B6C3F_1$	1:10 brei	ip
$CD8F_1$ mammary carcinoma[a]	$CD8F_1$	1:20 brei	sc
Colon 38 carcinoma	BDF_1, $B6C3F_1$	70 mg fragment	sc
L1210 leukemia	BDF_1, CDF_1	10^5 ascites cells	ip
P388 leukemia	BDF_1, CDF_1	10^6 ascites cells	ip
Lewis lung carcinoma	BDF_1, $B6C3D_1$	10^6 cells	iv
Human tumor xenografts			
CX-1 colon	nu/nu Swiss	1 x 1 x 1 mm fragment	src[b]
LX-1 lung	nu/nu Swiss	1 x 1 x 1 mm fragment	src[b]
MX-1 mammary	nu/nu Swiss	1 x 1 x 1 mm fragment	src[b]

[a] $CD8F_1$ mammary tumor tests are conducted in mice bearing the first transplant generation from the spontaneous tumor.

[b] Subrenal capsule.

Table 2

Tumor Panel Models: Treatment and Evaluation Factors

Model	Drug Route/ Schedule	Parameter	Active T/C (%)[a]		Evaluation Day
			MC1 (+)	DN2 (++)	
		Tumor Panel			
Mouse tumors					
ip B16 melanoma	ip/Q1D, D1-9	Median survival time	≥125	≥150	60
sc $CD8F_1$ mammary	ip/Q1D, once[b]	Median tumor weight change	≤20	≤0	30
sc Colon 38	ip/Q7D, D2-9	Median tumor weight change	≤42	≤10	20
iv Lewis lung	ip/Q1D, D1-9	Median survival time	≥140	≥150	60
ip L1210 leukemia	ip/Q1D, D1-9	Median survival time	≥125	≥150	30
Human tumor xenografts					
src CX-1 colon	sc/Q4D, D1-13	Mean tumor weight change	≤20	≤10	15
src LX-1 lung	sc/Q4D, D1-9	Mean tumor weight change	≤20	≤10	11
src MX-1 mammary	sc/Q4D, D1-9	Mean tumor weight change	≤20	≤10	11

a For survival assays, T/C is computed as survival time of treated mice x 100 ÷ survival time of controls. For tumor inhibition assays, T/C is computed as change in weight of treated tumor x 100 ÷ change in weight of control tumors.

b Treatment given when tumors reach weight of 100-700 mg.

considered a basis for selection priority even though it indicated a statistically significant difference from control behavior. The higher level of activity, DN2, was required for the selection of preclinical development candidates. The tumor panel system was designed both to detect agents with some tumor type "selectivity" (*i.e.*, activity in a single model) and to identify those with broad activity in many or all of the models. The goal was to decide which of the general screening procedures produced more clinically active compounds and to use such information to design antitumor screening programs. Another crucial question was whether there was any correlation between activity against a human tumor xenograft and a mouse tumor at the same site (*e.g.*, mouse colon tumor *vs.* human colon tumor), that is whether tumors of murine origin could be compared with the corresponding human tumors.

Result of the tumor panel approach. A detailed evaluation of results of tumor panel testing on 1085 compounds has been presented by Venditti *et al.*, who derived some cross-correlations among the animal models. Because clinical studies on the drugs selected for development based on the tumor panel testing are still incomplete, it is not yet possible to evaluate the approach. Nevertheless, the conclusions from the "tumor panel experiment" that seem clear thus far are as follows:

1. The sensitivities of the models to drugs appeared to parallel clinical experience in that the order of number of actives found by tumor site was leukemia > melanoma > mammary > lung > colon with very few actives being found in either the lung or colon models of either mouse (Lewis Lung, colon 38) or human (LX-1 lung, CX-1 colon xenografts) origin.
2. There was little correlation of activity by site between mouse and human tumors. While compounds active in the mouse mammary tumor showed more activity in the human mammary xenograft than a random sample of compounds, these same compounds similarly showed enhanced activity in most of the tumor panel models. This suggested that a compound having activity in any one tumor was much more likely to have activity in a second tumor than a randomly chosen compound.
3. Agents with substantial preclinical activity in animal solid tumors could be discovered which were inactive or marginally active against L1210 leukemia.
4. Some compounds found active against the human tumor xenografts, particularly the mammary xenograft, were inactive or marginally active against the mouse tumors in the panel.

It will be at least five to seven years before the tumor panel screening results can be correlated with the clinical effectiveness of the compounds selected. The outcome is inherently biased, however, by two factors; the use of a single (leukemia model) prescreen and the attempt to represent each tumor class by only one or two models. For example, there is no simple way to find out whether the one human lung tumor xenograft in the panel is representative of even a small percentage of human lung tumors. What is clear, is that, considering the wide diversity of tumor subtypes, potentially important leads may be missed unless the relevant and representative subtypes are part of the initial screens. Too many *in vivo* models would be required to have a comprehensive primary screen for agents active against the major human solid tumors (*e.g.*, lung, colon, breast). A new strategy is clearly needed to screen for agents against particular cancer types, that is, a "disease-oriented" screen.

DEVELOPMENT OF A NEW IN VITRO/IN VIVO HUMAN TUMOR-BASED "DISEASE-ORIENTED" DRUG SCREENING PROGRAM

The concept and the approach. As described above, the "compound-oriented" drug screening program conducted by the NCI was successful primarily in identifying compounds with clinical activity against leukemias and lymphomas. Many of these compounds are myelosuppressive and this may be related to the use of murine leukemia models as prescreens. In developing a "disease-oriented" approach to drug screening, it is essential that each compound be tested directly against a spectrum of tumor types without interposing a prescreen that could eliminate the very compounds of prime interest. Figure 3 shows a schematic representation of a new "disease-oriented" NCI drug screening program currently under development (for other background references, see refs. 5-8). Considering the known heterogeneity between and within histologic tumor types, this approach requires use of multiple representatives of each tumor type targeted in the "disease-oriented" strategy.

The screening of large numbers of unknown compounds using *in vivo* models rapidly becomes unmanageable and prohibitively expensive as multiple models are added. To meet this requirement efficiently the NCI has begun to develop human tumor cell line panels for primary *in vitro* screening. The approach is to develop panels of cell lines representative of particular tumor types and to test each unknown compound in all cell lines. As described more fully below, the object of this screening is to identify compounds which exert selective effects on particular tumor types and to follow these *in vitro* screening leads with *in vivo* testing, utilizing cell lines previously shown to be sensitive.

The screening models. Implementing this *in vitro/in vivo* "disease-oriented" screening program requires acquisition and characterization of tumor cell lines for construction of the cell line panels and development and validation of assay methods for *in vitro* and *in vivo* testing with these cell lines. In approaching this task, the highest initial priority has been given to constructing a representative cell line panel for lung cancer and to developing highly automated *in vitro* assay methods useful for these and other cell types. This "disease-oriented" program is now being developed, with further study and implementation planned for the next 2-3 years.

Beginning with the development of a lung cancer cell line panel, more than 20 cell lines representing squamous cell carcinoma, adenosquamous carcinoma, bronchioloalveolar carcinoma, large cell carcinoma, and "classic" and "variant" forms of small cell lung cancer have been acquired and extensively characterized. These lines have been subjected to careful scrutiny to ensure their freedom from adventitious agents (especially mycoplasma and murine hepatitis virus), and to verify their human origin (based on isoenzyme pattern and karyotype), the authentic histology of tumors produced in athymic mice, and their suitability for use in automated inhibition assays. Acquisition of additional cell lines for development of colon and other disease panels has recently begun.

Large-scale "disease-oriented" drug screening, even in an *in vitro* setting, requires highly efficient assay technology. Screening of 10,000 compounds per year in 60-90 cell lines requires more than 6-9 million cultures. A colorimetric assay (modified from Mosmann[9]) compatible with this volume of testing has been developed. The assay, which is performed in microculture plates, is based on reduction of a tetrazolium salt (MTT) to a colored formazan inside viable cells. Assay plates are read on a standard ELISA reader, which is interfaced to a computer for efficient data acquisition, storage, retrieval, and analysis. After testing in each cell line, compounds will be classified as showing statistically significant differential cytotoxicity or as lacking differential cytotoxicity. Compounds in the former category will be given the higher priority for development. Within this category, compounds showing selective cytotoxicity for particular tumor types will be assigned the highest priority. Indeed, the identification of these latter compounds is the major goal of the program. The *in vitro* screening leads will be subjected to *in vivo* testing using known sensitive cell lines. In parallel with the *in vivo* animal studies, compounds showing exquisite selectivity will be advanced promptly to toxicology studies and considered for expedited clinical trials, particularly in certain diseases, such as non small-cell lung cancer, for which no effective alternative treatment exists.

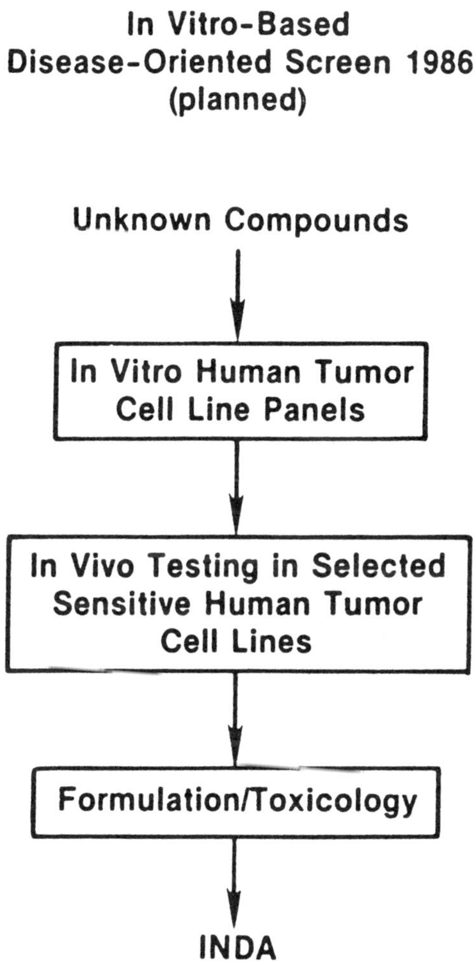
In Vitro-Based
Disease-Oriented Screen 1986
(planned)
Unknown Compounds
In Vitro Human Tumor Cell Line Panels
In Vivo Testing in Selected Sensitive Human Tumor Cell Lines
Formulation/Toxicology
INDA

Figure 3

The human tumor cell lines acquired for the lung cancer panel offer several possibilities for preclinical *in vivo* therapeutic trials. Most of the lines are highly tumorigenic in nude mice so that assays based on measurements of tumor mass may be performed. However, some of the cell lines grow very slowly, making these assays rather impractical. Subrenal capsule assays are also feasible for most of the lung cancer lines and offer the advantage of rapid turn-around time and reasonable cost. Several of the lines which manifest very aggressive growth in athymic mice, producing lethal disease and distant metastases, may allow useful preclinical therapeutic trials with survival as the endpoint. Other novel *in vivo* assays, which allow direct assessment of tumor growth and/or viability, are under development.

As described above, the development of this *in vitro/in vivo* "disease-oriented" drug screening program has been focused initially on lung cancer. Model development in this area has required approximately one year and pilot-scale screening will begin in early 1986. As indicated by the results of this screening, additional "disease-oriented" screening panels will be developed and the scale of the screening increased.

CHANGING PROSPECTS FOR NATURAL PRODUCTS RESEARCH

<u>Limitations of the former screening system of P388/tumor panel for natural products screening and isolation</u>. The L1210, P388, and the P388/tumor panel screens used from 1970 until 1984 revealed a variety of interesting new chemical structures active in one or more of these model systems. Once leads were discovered *in vivo*, fractionation was undertaken using either P388 or Eagle's KB cells *in vitro*. Unfortunately, materials obtained this way did not always give products with the expected *in vivo* activity; in some cases, the entire fractionation had to be done using costly and very time-consuming *in vivo* bioassays. Moreover, a very serious limitation resulted because many bioactive natural products occur at low concentrations and many leads were probably missed because the active constituent was not especially potent or the amounts were otherwise too small to detect. Most of the compounds advanced to clinical trials were active at 1 mg/kg/day or below in the P388 leukemia assay (*e.g.*, maytansine, camptothecin, bruceantin, and didemnin B), and it is quite likely that many novel compounds with possible antitumor activity remain undetected.

An approach utilizing primary *in vivo* screening thus may uncover mainly agents that are highly cytotoxic ("potent"), broadly active (generally cytotoxic), and present in substantial amounts. Moreover, because of these general selection criteria, there is a tendency repeatedly to "rediscover" these compounds. For example, toward the later stages of the NCI plant program from the mid-1970's through 1981, there were several re-isolations of camptothecin, maytansine, and bruceantin-related quassinoids. As more compounds with cancer-related activities are discovered from marine organisms, a similar situation might occur if there were a continuing primary reliance upon prescreens such as the P388 leukemia.

<u>Advantages of new *in vitro* screening models for natural products and tumor panel assays</u>. The new *in vitro* cell line screening panels present several new opportunities. Generally cytotoxic agents, some of which may have antitumor activity for fast-growing tumors, will not be missed since such agents will demonstrate toxicity towards many of the cell lines. Additionally and most importantly, there will be the opportunity to find highly tumor-type selective (and probably rare) compounds; this is the ultimate goal of the new program.

The *in vitro* cell line screen is at least 100 times more sensitive than a primary *in vivo* screen, as estimated by conversion of the drug concentration required for 50% inhibition of cell growth in culture to the drug dosage (mg/kg) needed to achieve that concentration in the body (μg/mL of body fluid, assuming rapid distribution and no metabolic loss). The enhanced sensitivity of the screens will allow discovery of less "potent" substances and substances present at low concentrations. The bioassay-directed isolation of selectively cytotoxic major components will utilize one or more of the cell lines found to be sensitive in the initial screening. Isolation procedures may be hastened by the use of a highly discriminating *in vitro* bioassay, but a specific bioassay must be readily available. It is expected that, instead of having all cell lines continuously on hand, groups of cell lines will be rotated to maximize testing and minimize cross-contamination. Computerized scheduling can be used to give priority at a particular time to screening with cell lines which are also in use as bioassays to guide fractionation.

Aside from the major technical advantages offered by the new screens, the most important advantage of the use of cell line batteries is the possibility for discovery of tumor-type specific compounds. Such compounds will probably be of novel chemo- and/or biotypes not even detectable by the prior screens. Clearly, natural products will play a pivotal role in the NCI's exploration of the concept of tumor-type-specific compounds for treatment of human solid tumors.

THE POTENTIAL OF THE SEA AS A SOURCE OF NEW ANTICANCER SUBSTANCES

The potential of the marine environment as a source of novel drugs is only beginning to be realized, though indications of this potential were obtained as early as 1955 with the isolation of the biologically active nucleosides, spongouridine (1), spongothymidine (2), and spongosine (3), from the sponge *Cryptotethya crypta*[10,11]. These compounds led, 20 years later, to the development of adenine arabinoside and the clinically useful anticancer drug, cytosine arabinoside (Ara-A and Ara-C, respectively).

In the past 20 years the NCI has screened over 18,000 extracts of marine organisms, mainly using the *in vivo* P388 model as the primary screen. A great variety of novel structure types exhibiting varying degrees of *in vivo* activity and/or cytotoxicity have been isolated, and a number of promising leads have been discovered. One of these, didemnin B (4), isolated from the tunicate *Trididemnum* sp.,[12] is currently undergoing clinical trials.

Other biologically active cyclic peptides have been isolated from tunicate species; *Lissoclinum patella* yielded the cytotoxic patellamides A, B (5), and C (6), together with the novel disulfide-bridged analogue, ulithiacyclamide (7).[13-16] In addition, bioassay-directed fractionation of extracts of a sea hare, *Dollabella auricularia*, resulted in the isolation of a number of similar cyclic peptides, the dolastatins, some of which possess promising antitumor activity.[17] The fistularins [*e.g.*, fistularin-3 (8)] isolated from the sponge *Aplysina fistularis* forma *fulva*, further exemplify novel nitrogen-containing metabolites isolated from marine sources.[18] These compounds all possess marked cytotoxicity.

The macrocyclic polyether lactones, the bryostatins, isolated from the bryozoan *Bugula neritina*,[19,20] exhibit potent activity in the P388 mouse leukemia system, and also strongly affect the activity of protein kinase C, a kinase shown to influence strongly the proliferation of tumor cells.[21] The structure of bryostatin 1 (9) was confirmed by X-ray crystallographic analysis,[19] and the structures of the other bryostatins have been elucidated by comparison of H-NMR data with those for 9.

Unusual macrocyclic lactones have also been isolated from the eggmasses of nudibranches. Ulapualides A (10) and B from the eggs of *Hexabranchus sanguineus* are strong inhibitors of L1210 leukemia cell proliferation and might be responsible for the virtual immunity of such eggmasses to predation,[22] while a closely related macrolide, kabiramide C, isolated from the eggs of an unidentified nudibranch collected at Kabira Bay in the Ryukyu Islands, possesses antifungal activity.[23] The structure of the novel cyto-

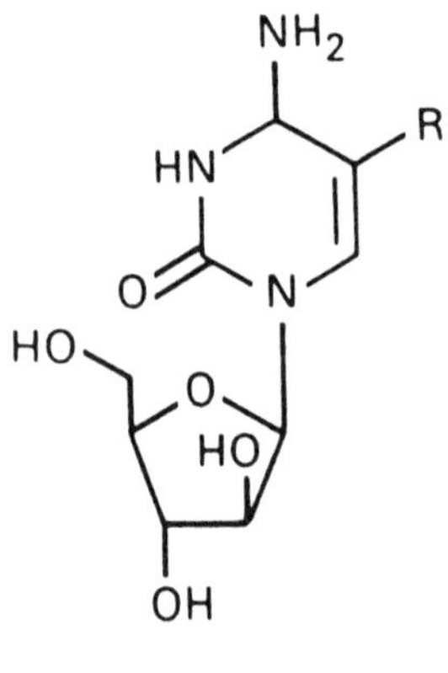

1 R = H

2 R = CH_3

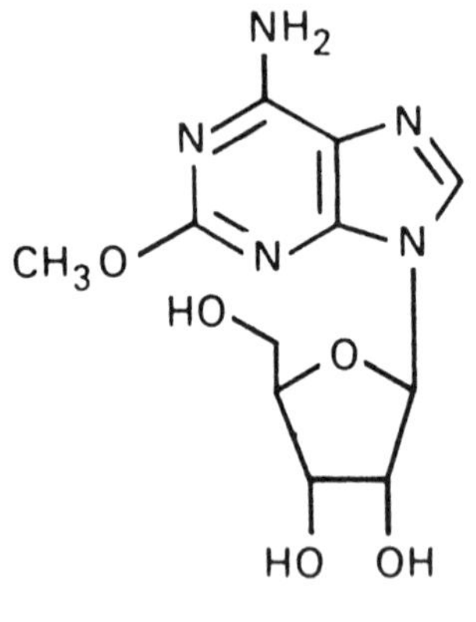

3

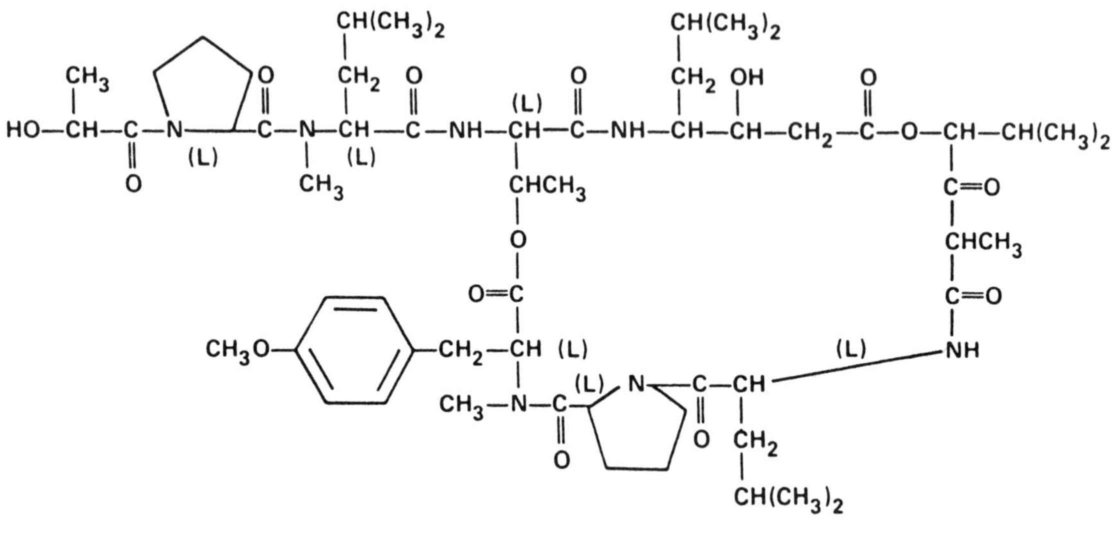

4

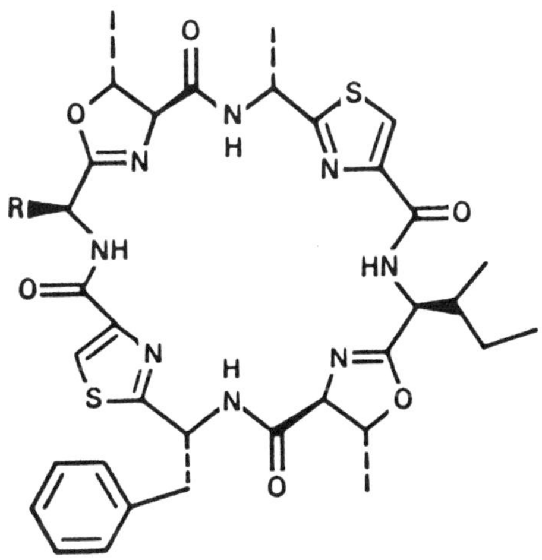

5 R = $(CH_3)_2CHCH_2$

6 R = $(CH_3)_2CH$

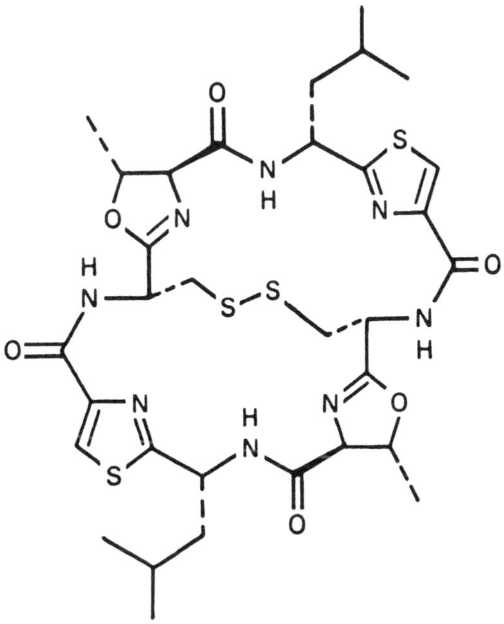

7

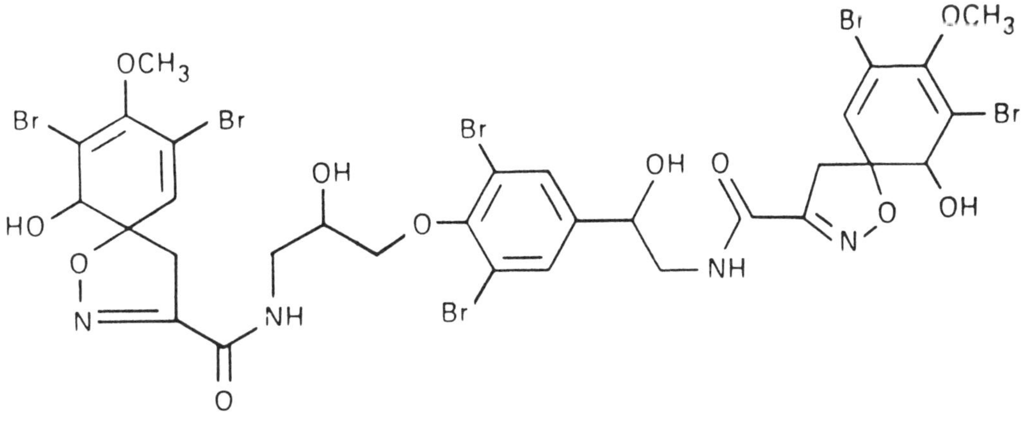

8

toxic episulfide-containing polyether, acanthifolicin (11), isolated from the sponge *Pandaros acanthifolium*, was established by X-ray crystallography.[24] Gorgonians are noteworthy as the source of a number of prostaglandins.[25] The isolation of a novel series of physiologically active eicosanoids from the coral, *Telesto riisei*, has recently been reported.[26] One of these compounds, the chlorinated metabolite punaglandin-3 (12), exhibits strong *in vitro* activity in the L1210 leukemia system. An unusual cytotoxic diterpene, spatol (13), has been isolated from the brown alga, *Spatoglossum schmittii*.[27] In recent years blue-green algae have received increasing attention as sources of new potential anticancer agents.[28] Debromoaplysiatoxin (14) has been shown to be the major antineoplastic constituent of *Lyngbya majuscula*,[29] while it and a closely related compound, oscillatoxin A (15), were identified as the antineoplastic constituents of an extract of a mixture of two cyanophytes tentatively identified as *Schizothrix calcicola* and *Oscillatoria nigroviridis*.[30] It is interesting to note that 14 has also been isolated from the digestive gland of the sea hare, *Stylocheilus longicauda*, which has been observed feeding on *L. majuscula*,[31] thereby providing convincing evidence that some marine organisms metabolites can be of dietary origin. Two other active macrocyclic lactones, acutiphycin (16) and 20,21-didehydroacutiphycin (17), have recently been isolated from *Oscillatoria acutissima*.[32]

New areas of emphasis for marine biological investigations by the NCI. The marine environment remains relatively unexplored as a source of new drugs, but its potential in this respect is clearly apparent from the variety of biologically active compounds of novel structural types isolated in recent years, as illustrated above. These observations, together with the introduction of the "disease-oriented" primary screen, prompted the NCI to promote the investigation of marine organisms as a major source of selective anticancer agents.

Shallow-water and deep-water collections. The extracts screened by the NCI thus far have been mainly from shallow-water organisms submitted voluntarily by marine natural product chemists worldwide. An extensive new shallow-water collection program in the Indo-Pacific will be initiated by the NCI in late 1986, at the same time that a deep-water collection project begins. To date, relatively few organisms have been collected at depths greater than 100 feet, and it seems likely that the differences between shallow- and deep-water organisms will be reflected in their diverse biological activities. The new collection programs are designed to obtain approximately 15,000 marine organisms over a five-year period in quantities sufficient to provide extracts suitable for testing in the "disease-oriented" primary screen and in new screens as they become available. These marine organisms and approximately 20,000 plants to be collected in rain forests during the next five years will be extracted (organic and aqueous) at an NCI-designated facility and the extracts will be stored at low temperatures in a sample repository near the screening laboratories. Organisms yielding active extracts will be re-collected on a larger scale in order to proceed with the isolation and characterization of the active components. All organisms collected will be thoroughly documented and identified, and preserved specimens will be deposited in a national facility.

Marine fermentations. As noted earlier, a number of novel active compounds have been isolated from blue-green algae. In addition, the antitumor activity of certain sponges and mosses has been correlated with their association with microflora, including blue-green algae, and it is clear that these microalgae merit intensive investigation. Therefore, in late 1986, the NCI will initiate a five-year project aimed at the isolation and cultivation of 1,000 blue-green algae from a variety of marine and terrestrial sources. Organic solvent and aqueous cell extracts will be provided to the NCI for low-temperature storage in the sample repository and testing in the "disease-oriented", and in future new screens. Active cultures will be optimized and regrown to provide sufficient material for the isolation and characterization of active constituents, and all cultures will be suitably

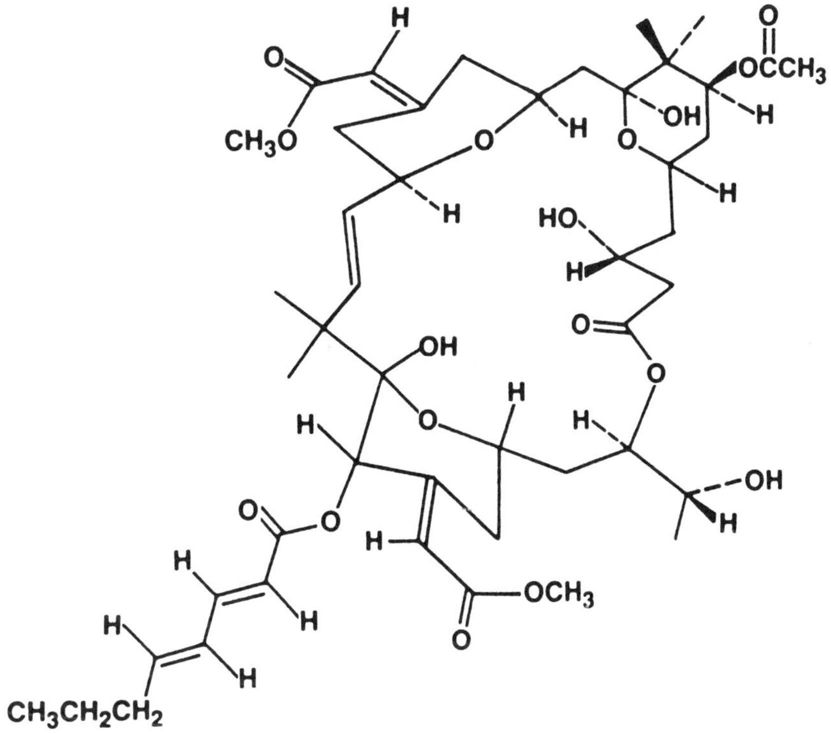

9

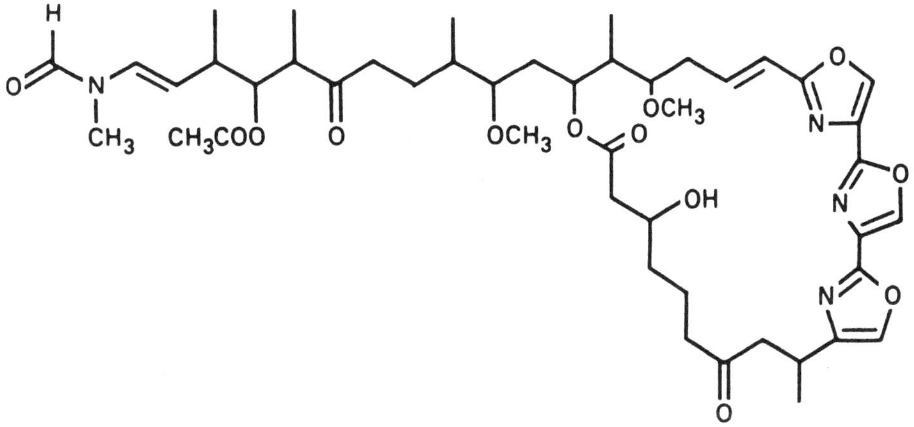

10

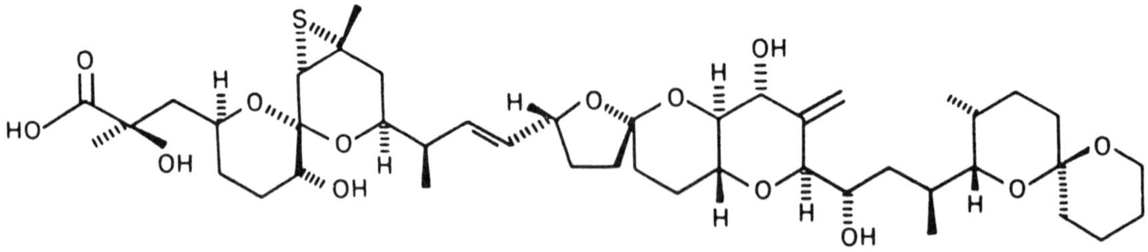

11

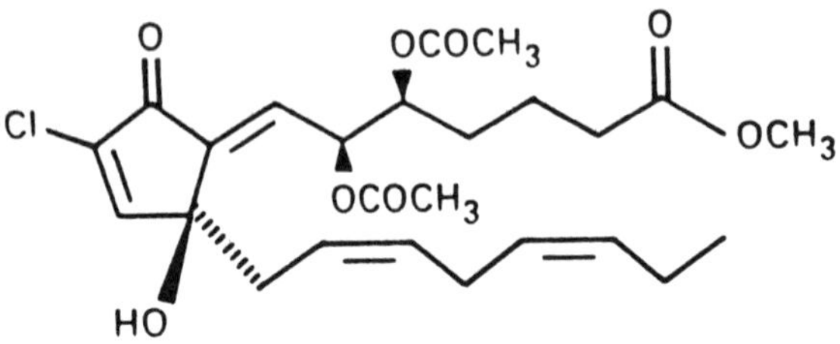

12

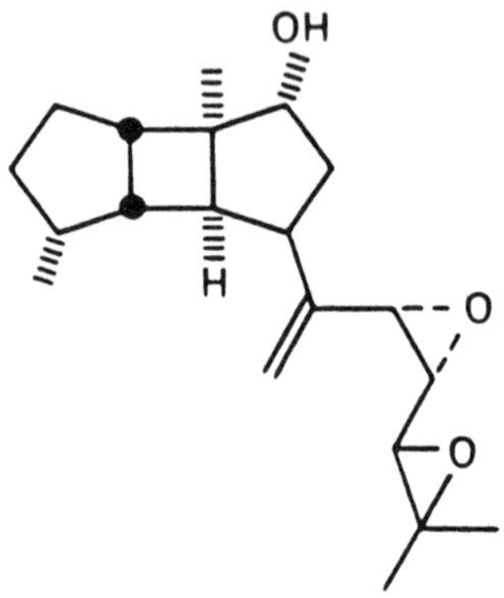

13

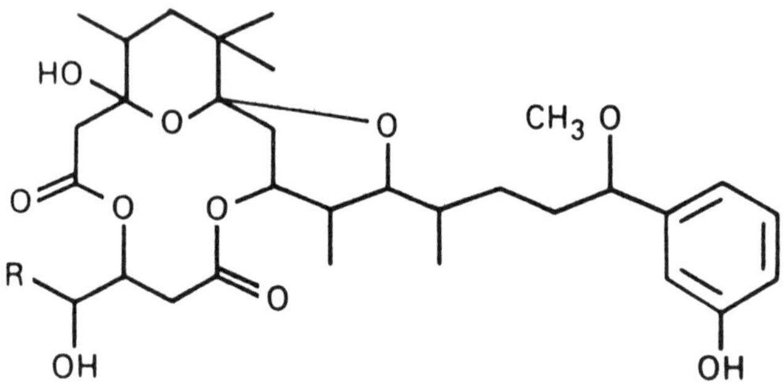

14 R = CH_3

15 R = H

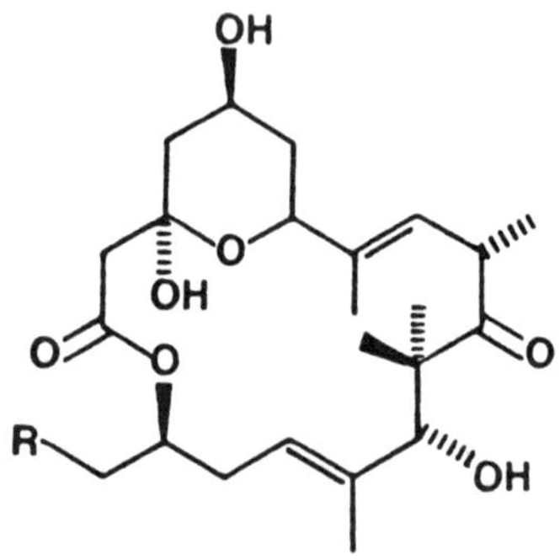

16 R = $CH_3CH_2CH_2CH_2$

17 R = 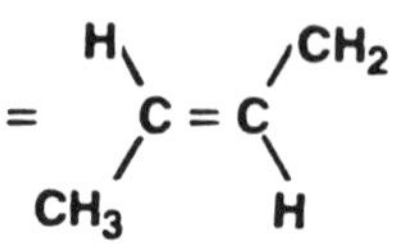

preserved and stored in an appropriate facility. The potential of marine microorganisms as sources of novel anticancer agents will also be explored over a five-year period to provide extracts of approximately 1,500 cultures.

SUMMARY AND PERSPECTIVE

A shift in the NCI drug discovery program toward a specific "disease-oriented" strategy is intended to offer new opportunities for the discovery of novel drug candidates with potential activity against the major human cancers, which have thus far eluded effective treatment. The new screening program should particularly facilitate the detection, isolation, and identification of new kinds of leads from natural products. The enhanced sensitivity and selectivity of the *in vitro* human tumor cell line panels as the primary screen will reveal new natural products for intensive investigation. The relatively unexplored marine area appears especially promising. The new marine natural products acquisition projects of the NCI will function in concert with the new screening project to open new and productive avenues for the investigation of marine biologicals.

REFERENCES

1. Goldin, A; Sepick, A.A.; Mantel, N., *Cancer Chemother. Rep.*, 1966, *50*, 173.
2. Goldin, A.; Schepartz, S.A.; Venditti, J.M.; DeVita, V.T., Jr., *Methods Cancer Res.*, 1979, *16A*, 165.
3. Johnson, R.K.; Goldin, A., *Cancer Treat. Rev.*, 1975, *2*, 1.
4. Venditti, J.M.; Wesley, R.A.; Plowman, J., *Adv. Pharmacol. Chemother.*, 1984, *20*, 1.
5. Boyd, M.R.; in Frei, E.J. and Freireich, E.J., Eds., *Cancer Therapy: Where Do We Go From Here?*, Proceedings of the General Motors Cancer Research Foundation Conference, Jackson Hole, Wyoming, September 14-15, 1984. Lippincott, in press.
6. Boyd, M.R.; NIH new drug program. *Fourth World Conference on Lung Cancer: Mini Symposia Proceedings*, Toronto, Canada, August 25-30, 1985.
7. Boyd, M.R.; McLemore, T.; Johnston, M.; Gazdar, A.; Minna, J.; Shoemaker, R., in J.A. Roth; J.C. Ruckdeschel; T.H. Weisenburger, Eds., *Thoracic Oncology*, W.B. Saunders Co, New York, NY, chap 51.
8. "NCI planning to switch drug development emphasis from compound to human cancer-oriented strategy", *Cancer Lett.*, 1984, *10*, 1.
9. Mosmann, T., *J. Immunol. Methods*, 1983, *65*, 55.
10. Bergmann, W.; Burke, D.C., *J. Org. Chem.*, 1955, *20*, 1501.
11. Bergmann, W.; Burke, D.C., *J. Org. Chem.*, 1956, *21*, 226.
12. Rinehart, K.L., Jr.; Gloer, J.B.; Cook, J.C.; Mizsak, S.A.; Scahill, T.A., *J. Am. Chem. Soc.*, 1981, *103*, 1857.
13. Hamada, M.; Shibata, M.; Shioiri, T., *Tetrahedron Lett.*, 1985, *26*, 5155, 5159.
14. Sesin, D.F.; Gaskell, S.J.; Ireland, C.M., *Bull. Soc. Chim. Belge*, 1986, in press.
15. Wasylyk, J.M.; Biskupiak, J.E.; Costello, C.E.; Ireland, C.M., *J. Org. Chem.*, 1983, *48*, 4445.
16. Ireland, C.M.; Durso, A.R., Jr.; Newman, R.A.; Hacker, M.P., *J. Org. Chem.*, 1982, *47*, 1807.
17. Pettit, G.R.; Kamano, Y.; Brown, P.; Gust, D.; Inoue, M.; Herald, C.L., *J. Am. Chem. Soc.*, 1982, *104*, 905.
18. Gopichand, Y.; Schmitz, F.J., *Tetrahedron Lett.*, 1979, 3921.
19. Pettit, G.R.; Herald, C.L.; Doubek, D.L.; Herald, D.L.; Arnold, E.; Clardy, J., *J. Am. Chem. Soc.*, 1982, *104*, 6846.
20. Pettit, G.R.; Kamano, Y.; Herald, C.L.; Tozawa, M., *Can. J. Chem.*, 1985, *63*, 1204.

21. Smith, J.B.; Smith, L.; Pettit, G.R., *Biochem. Biophys. Res. Commun.*, 1985, *132*, 939.
22. Roesener, J.A.; Scheuer, P.J., *J. Am. Chem. Soc.*, 1986, *108*, 846.
23. Matsunaga, S.; Fusetani, N.; Hashimoto, K.; Koseki, K.; Noma, M., *J. Am. Chem. Soc.*, 1986, *108*, 847.
24. Schmitz, F.J.; Prasad, R.S.; Gopichand, Y.; Hossain, M.B.; van der Helm, D.; Schmidt, P., *J. Am. Chem. Soc.*, 1981, *103*, 2467.
25. Weinheimer, A.J.; Spraggins, R.L., *Tetrahedron Lett.*, 1969, 5185.
26. Baker, B.J.; Okuda, R.K.; Yu, P.T.K.; Scheuer, P.J., *J. Am. Chem. Soc.*, 1985, *107*, 2976.
27. Gerwick, W.H.; Fenical, W.; van Engen, D.; Clardy, J., *J. Am. Chem. Soc.*, 1980, *102*, 7991.
28. Moore, R.E., *Pure Appl. Chem.*, 1982, *54*, 1919.
29. Mynderse, J.S.; Moore, R.E.; Kashiwagi, M.; Norton, T.R., *Science (Washington, D.C.)*, 1977, *196*, 538.
30. Mynderse, J.S.; Moore, R.E., *J. Org. Chem.*, 1978, *43*, 2301.
31. Kato, Y.; Scheuer, P., *Pure Appl. Chem.*, 1975, *41*, 1.
32. Barchi, J.J.; Moore, R.E.; Patterson, G.M.L., *J. Am. Chem. Soc.*, 1984, *106*, 8193.

Gary L. Neil
Therapeutics Reasearch, The Upjohn Company, Kalamazoo, Michigan 49001, U.S.A.

Medical Needs and the Pharmaceutical Market

A general review of current needs for new pharmaceutical agents in various therapeutic fields--for new antimicrobial, antiviral, and antineoplastic agents, for cardioregulators, immunomodulators, and other agents in both human and animal medicine--will be presented here and in Dr. Delappe's remarks elsewhere in this book. While attention must surely be directed to the need for improved antiinfective agents, for anticancer drugs, and for immunomodulators, I shall begin with a broad review of the need for new pharmaceutical agents and shall describe first the background against which that need is set, the current worldwide pharmaceutical market.

It must be noted that if a new agent derived from a marine organism collected this weekend were developed successfully, it would cost more than $70 million* and not reach the major markets and be widely used before the end of this century. If there was an acute use indication, then the process could be shortened by 2-3 years. The important factor, then, is not today's market but the market as we expect it to be in the late 1990's.[1] That future market is likely to be defined largely by our ability to meet medical needs that are not met in the present market, that is, our ability to close the so-called "therapeutic gap". The many important factors to be considered if confidence is to be placed in predictions about the market will not be reviewed in any detail here, but I shall define the important medical needs which are likely to remain at the end of this century and examine some demographic trends which will result, by that time, in the attachment of greater importance to certain current medical needs.

CURRENT WORLDWIDE PHARMACEUTICAL MARKET

In recently released figures,[2] IMS International estimates the 1984 world pharmaceutical market at *ca.* $87 billion. This represents a modest 2% growth from 1983, due primarily to the continued strength of the U.S. dollar and an actual decline in the Japanese market as a result of increasingly stringent price controls by the Japanese government. The United States and Canada continue to dominate as the largest segment (30%) with the Africa/Asia/Australia segment second (26%) and Europe close behind (23%). The 16 top countries accounted for *ca.* 84% of free-world sales with the United States still leading

---

*All figures are given in United States dollars.

(24.2 billion), followed by Japan (13.0 billion) and W. Germany (5.4 billion). Only three other countries have pharmaceutical markets in excess of 2 billion.

Examination of *per capita* pharmaceutical consumption represents another interesting way to examine the worldwide pharmaceutical market. Based on 1976 figures,[3] Japan ranked first $95 *per capita*. The USA was only sixth $70 *per capita*, with eight European countries filling out the top ten. In 1973, overall world drug sales represented $7.5 *per capita* with Japan highest at $49. Developed countries consumed an average $23 *per capita* with developing countries able to afford only $3 per person. The Indian pharmaceutical market, which now ranks 11th in total market worldwide at *ca.* 1 billion, was estimated to be $0.80 per person in 1973.

The six largest therapeutic categories[2] accounted for about 75% of 1984 worldwide audited sales. They were, in order: alimentary tract and metabolic disorder treatments, including antiulcer, antidiabetic agents and vitamins; cardiovasculars including calcium antagonists, nitrates, antiarrhythmics, beta blockers, peripheral vasodilators, and diuretics; antiinfectives, including systemic antibiotics, vaccines, systemic antifungals, and antivirals; central nervous system drugs, including analgesics, psycholeptics, psychoanaleptics, antiepileptics, and anaesthetics; respiratory tract drugs, particularly cough and cold preparations and asthmatics; musculoskeletal drugs, especially antirheumatics and muscle relaxants.

Estimates of the 1984 pharmaceutical market should be seen as a rough measure of what is possible today in meeting worldwide medical needs. I think that these data are of relatively limited value in helping us select areas of emphasis for research efforts. Indeed, it would seem advisable to concentrate on those obvious medical needs that are likely to be unmet in the next 10-20 years even though the current market for those areas may be relatively small. Accordingly, a focus on diseases such as cancer and viral infections would seem appropriate with, however, a word of caution. The choice 10-15 years ago of such a strategy might have led one to avoid new antibiotics as a therapeutic goal. Based on the market at that time and an assessment of unmet medical needs, one could easily have concluded that new antibiotics represented a relatively unattractive area. In fact, new antibiotics have been eagerly accepted in the market and that area continues to show healthy growth. Clearly then, the strategies we adopt must be tempered by a careful assessment of other factors, including the probability of achieving the set goals. When the goal is an antibiotic with certain advantages over those already available, the chances of success are clearly greater than if the goal were to cure cancer.

UNMET MEDICAL NEEDS

On a worldwide basis, one realizes immediately that medical needs in developed, industrialized, and relatively wealthy nations are markedly different from those in the developing, low-income world. In developing countries, reliable, accurate data comparable to that available for most developed nations are extremely difficult to obtain, even on the causes of mortality and morbidity. However, the differences in life expectancy, birth rate, and death rate are enormous and indicate clearly our inability to meet the health needs of the people in underdeveloped nations.

In a 1975 survey, the U.S. Pharmaceutical Manufacturing Association compared the pharmaceutical market of 34 low-income countries (including *ca.* 1/3 of the world's population with $150 *per capita* gross national product) with that of 19 industrialized countries (17% of the world's population with $6200 *per capita* gross national product).[4] It would appear to be no coincidence that the *per capita* pharmaceutical consumption of the low-income countries (with life expectancies not much more than 60% of those in the industrialized countries and with birth and death rates three times and two times those of the industrialized countries, respectively) was less than 3% of that of more fortunate countries. Clearly, much of the unmet medical need is unrelated to scientific and medical factors but instead is determined by social, political, and especially by economic considerations. A comparison of the causes of death in various parts of the world emphasizes this conclusion even though accurate data are difficult to obtain. Microbial infection has been almost eliminated as a major cause of death in the U.S., but it continues to take a huge toll in the underdeveloped world and even in the so-called "middle income" countries.

This analysis, however, is too simplistic and superficial. Certain infectious diseases, particularly those transmitted by parasites, are endemic to large portions of the underdeveloped nations. Malaria, a disease which we had reason to believe had been brought under control 20 years ago, today afflicts 200-400 million people. In Africa, it kills 10% of its victims and debilitates the rest, and in some areas it accounts for 50% of childhood mortality. Other tropical parasitic diseases are equally devastating. Fifty million people are estimated to be at direct risk of contracting trypanosomiasis, a fatal neurological disease finally manifesting itself in humans as sleeping sickness. There is little doubt that the control of these and related diseases would have an enormous impact on both human life expectancy and the quality of life. Even the cure of cancer would probably pale in comparison. In spite of this obvious medical need, relatively little effort has been devoted to pharmaceutical control of these enormous health problems. Again, political, social, and, particularly, economic considerations are dominant. It is interesting to note that much progress in the treatment of parasitic diseases derives not from human health research but from efforts to control similar infections in food-producing animals; this somewhat tragic irony nevertheless offers hope for millions of people.

Let's consider now the medical needs in the developed nations, that is, those areas where an economic return on a research investment might be likely. Those diseases and conditions which cause major loss of life represent obvious targets for research. In the United States in 1975 those diseases were, in order: heart disease, cancer, cerebrovascular disease, trauma (accidents), influenza and pneumonia, diabetes, cirrhosis of the liver, and arteriosclerosis.[5] In contrast, in 1900, influenza and pneumonia led the list, with tuberculosis close behind. Diarrhea and enteritis were as important as heart disease, and cancer was not in the top five. This change is a strong testament to the preeminent contribution of pharmaceutical research in this century, the antibiotic.

What will be the impact on life expectancy of the development of successful therapy for either of the current major killers, heart disease and cancer? Surprisingly, the complete elimination of cancer as a cause of death would add only *ca.* 2.5 years to life expectancy at birth, the elimination of cardiovascular diseases would add 12.4 years.[6] The life expectancy of an individual would be increased by less, 0.9 and 1.5 years respectively, for the two diseases. Clearly, deaths from these degenerative diseases occur largely in the advanced years of life. I do not wish to imply that the search for the cure or prevention of cancer or heart disease is an unworthy task; obviously it is important. We should, however, begin to think more in terms of adding life to years, than of adding years to life.

IMPROVED QUALITY OF LIFE AS A PHARMACEUTICAL GOAL

It is estimated that, by the year 2000, the number of individuals older than 65 years in the United States will have increased by 50%, from the present 24 million to 36 million, accounting for 14% of the population instead of the present 11%. In his excellent review, "Pharmaceuticals in the Year 2000",[5] P. Goldschmidt concludes that life expectancy in the United States is unlikely to increase significantly during the next 20 years. He suggests that the most important advances during that time will be improvement in the health and functional abilities of those who are alive. The elderly are now, and will be then, most affected by the major causes of disability and morbidity. In 1975 these were, in order: arthritis and rheumatism, heart conditions, visual impairments, hypertension, diabetes, and mental and nervous disorders.[5] Such diseases and conditions should, therefore, be the goals for therapeutic intervention as we seek new pharmaceuticals from all sources, including the sea. We need anthiarthritics (especially disease-modifying drugs), analgesics, antihypertensives, antiarrhythmic agents, antianginal drugs, antiobesity agents, antidepressants and anxiolytics, agents for the treatment of Alzheimer's disease, and agents to treat the sequelae of diabetes.

CONCLUSIONS

In another chapter of this book, the primary therapeutic targets of current research at SeaPharm, the leading company in marine-derived pharmaceuticals, are identified as anticancer, antiviral, antifungal, immunomodulatory, and cardiotonic agents. With the possible exception of cardiotonic agents, these targets are similar to those of companies involved in the traditional search for pharmaceutical agents from natural sources, in particular those produced by microorganisms under fermentation conditions, an area in which we at Upjohn have considerable experience.

SeaPharm's choice of therapeutic targets, like ours for fermentation-derived substances, may be determined more by the availability of high-volume *in vitro* detection systems which are reliable, predictive, sensitive, quantitative, quick, and inexpensive than by a comprehensive assessment of medical needs and the anticipated pharmaceutical market. Such technology is a *sine qua non* for natural products research. I would suggest, however, that given the rapid development of lead-finding technology in pharmaceutical research, based largely on recent advances in molecular and cellular biology, the stage is set to broaden greatly the search for therapeutically relevant bioactive compounds elaborated by natural sources. As diseases become better defined targets for therapeutic action at the molecular level will become more apparent. With those insights, I am certain that a broad range of new detection and assay systems suitable for the search for naturally derived therapeutic entities will become available. I believe the outlook for natural products as therapeutic entities has never been brighter and I am confident that such agents, including those from marine sources, will assume even more important roles in the pharmaceutical armamentarium of the future.

REFERENCES

1. Pharmaceuticals in the Year 2000. The Changing Context for Drug R&D, Clement Bezold, Ed., Institute for Alternative Futures, 1983.
2. D.A. West, I.M.S. International, quoted in Scrip, October 9, 1985.
3. The World Health Market. David Tucker, Facts on File Publications, New York, 1984.
4. The Pharmaceutical Industry and the Third World, Pharmaceutical Manufactures Association, Washington, D.C., 1979.
5. Peter G. Goldschmidt, Health Conditions in the Year 2000, pp 25-64, in Ref. 1.
6. Tsay, S.P.; Lee, E.S.; Hardy, R.J., *Am. J. Public Health*, 1978, 966.

Jere E. Goyan
School of Pharmacy, University of California, San Francisco, California 94143, U.S.A.

FDA Hurdles for the Development of New Marine Compounds

This discussion will deal with potential new prescription drugs, not with over-the-counter drugs, food additives, etc., and might well begin with a comment about its title. The term "hurdles" has, at least to me, the connotation that FDA has installed some obstacles to delay a sponsor in his "dash" to make new wonder drugs available to the public. Those who have had the opportunity to serve as commissioner of the Food and Drug Administration would argue that, although these requirements may slow the pace of the race, that is not their intended purpose. They are there to protect the public from what Peter Medawar has described as a "kindly conspiracy in which everybody has the very best intentions, the patient wants to get well, his physician wants to have made him better, and the pharmaceutical company would like to have put it into the physician's power to have made him so." The regulatory barriers that we wish to discuss were put in place to deal with this "kindly conspiracy".

In talking with groups of scientists unfamiliar with the arcane subject of the FD&C Act, I have always found it worthwhile to present a short history of the present Act. Back about the turn of the century, there were only a handful of effective drugs and literally thousands of nostrums. A typical example is Humbug Oil which, the labels notes, "cures diphtheria". Concern over the bilking of the public by such outlandish products and the adulteration of food, as revealed in Upton Sinclair's book, *The Jungle*, led to public outrage followed by congressional action with the passage of the 1906 Pure Food and Drug Act. It was the first attempt at regulation of the drug industry (although vaccines had come under such regulation a few years earlier) but only in a very mild fashion. Basically, it required that all such products disclose their contents on the label. The purveyors of such "remedies" quickly found a way of turning the labeling requirement to their own benefit by adding to the label the terminology, "guaranteed under the 1906 Pure Food and Drug Act", implying that the therapeutic claims were endorsed by the federal government. Although many attempts were made to change the law subsequent to that time, they were all vigorously opposed by the industry and successfully "beaten back" until 1938. There were approximately 100 victims of the "sulfanilamide elixir" disaster of 1937. Unfortunately, the elixir had been prepared using diethylene glycol, and although a pharmaceutically elegant and tasty product, it was also a deadly poison. The outcome again was public outrage followed by congressional action. The 1938 Pure Food, Drug and Cosmetic Act included a number of added requirements, the most important of which was that in the future all drugs had to be proven to be "safe". Obviously, the term safe is a relative one, but the requirement of the law resulted in regulations relative to appropriate testing in laboratory animals to determine LD_{50}s, etc., before such drugs might be tested in humans.

Again, although concern was expressed from time to time about some of the misuses of drugs in the United States and their potential to cause harm as well as good, no major changes in the Act occurred relative to drugs until 1962. That change was again the result of a drug tragedy. Most of you will remember that it was in that year that we became aware of the fact that the sedative-hypnotic thalidomide had been responsible for the birth of a large number of infants with phocomelia throughout the world, but only a few in the United States. Dr. Frances Kelsey received the Medal of Honor from then-President John F. Kennedy for her part in refusing to allow approval of thalidomide in the United States. Public outrage led to the passage of the first significant amendments relative to drugs in the FD&C Act. These 1962 amendments included the so-called efficacy requirement--that all drugs must be shown to work for the indication for which they are proposed. That requirement was at least partially brought about by concern that thalidomide samples had been sent to physicians throughout the United States, even though it had not been approved, so that individual physicians could run their own "study" of the usefulness of the drug. Such practices were common at that time, and obviously were an effective device to promote a new product.

Perhaps it is worthwhile to quote the legal language of the law relative to drug approval. If the Secretary of Health and Human Services finds that "(1) the investigations, reports of which are required to be submitted to the Secretary... do not include adequate tests by all methods reasonably applicable to show whether or not such drug is safe for use under the conditions prescribed, recommended, or suggested in the proposed labeling thereof; (2) the results of such tests show that such drug is unsafe for use under such conditions or do not show that such drug is safe for use under such conditions; (3) the methods used in, and the facilities and controls used for, the manufacture, processing, and packing of such drug are inadequate to preserve its identity, strength, quality, and purity; (4) upon the basis of the information submitted to him as part of the application, or upon the basis of any other information before him with respect to such drug, he has insufficient information to determine whether such drug is safe for use under such conditions; or (5) evaluated on the basis of the information submitted to him as part of the application and any other information before him with respect to such drug, there is a lack of substantial evidence that the drug will have the effect it purports or is represented to have under the conditions of use prescribed, recommended, or suggested in the proposed labeling thereof; or (6) based on a fair evaluation of all material facts, such labeling is false or misleading in any particular; he shall issue an order refusing to approve the application. If, after such notice and opportunity for hearing, the Secretary finds that clauses (1) through (6) do not apply, he shall issue an order approving the application. As used in this subsection... the term "substantial evidence" means evidence consisting of adequate and well-controlled investigations, including clinical investigations, by experts qualified by scientific training and experience to evaluate the effectiveness of the drug involved, on the basis of which it could fairly and responsibly be concluded by such experts that the drug will have the effect it purports or is represented to have under the conditions of use prescribed, recommended, or suggested in the labeling or proposed labeling thereof". That rather complex language, which requires that the drug be properly manufactured, properly labeled, and demonstrated to be safe and effective under the conditions of use, is the legal basis for all the regulations relative to the approval of new drugs. To my way of thinking there is no way that drugs derived from marine sources would be treated in any other fashion. Although there are constant attempts to provide additional guidelines and to update specific aspects of the IND/NDA process, the general scheme remains unchanged. It has been elucidated by the Agency over a period of years through notice and comment rule-making, as required by the Administrative Procedure Act.

In broad form, the scheme is as follows. Appropriate tests are done first on animals as an indication of whether the drug would be safe for humans. If such is the case, then the sponsor applies for an investigational new drug (IND) exemption, which allows him to administer the drug to humans. Phase I testing consists of safety tests of the drug in a small number of healthy volunteers and is sometimes referred to as the clinical pharmacology stage; it also establishes the range of dosages which may be tolerated by humans without toxicity. These short-term tests are, however, unlikely to reveal chronic toxicities.

When the drug has been shown to be relatively non-toxic, the sponsor moves to Phase II studies on individuals suffering from the disease that the drug is supposed to ameliorate or control. A drug useful in hypertension, for example, would be tested on a small group of hypertensive patients. If Phase II investigations are successful, the sponsor begins full-scale Phase III clinical testing on humans, involving a much larger group of patients.

The numbers of patients are usually determined by statistical evaluation, balancing the need to establish as firmly as possible the usefulness of the drug against the often immense cost of the studies. Thus, the Type I error is ordinarily set at 0.05, thereby establishing that a difference between treatments could occur, by chance, only once in 20 such trials, but the Type II error, the odds of the treatment showing no difference when one actually exists, are set higher. These studies are usually double blind; neither the investigator giving the drug nor the patient knows whether the drug, a placebo, or perhaps a positive control drug is being given.

This is the standard approach which meets the statutory requirement for substantial evidence as described. Assuming that the drug is thus found to be both safe and effective, the sponsor then makes application to market the drug with an appropriately prepared new drug application (NDA).

Both safety and efficacy are, to some degree, relative terms. No drug is completely safe nor effective in every patient. Thus, the FDA has to determine whether "under the conditions of use" the adverse effects to be expected will be tolerable considering the probable benefits. As an example, the Agency is always willing to approve a relatively toxic drug for an indication for which there is no effective medication or for which the new drug is significantly more effective than previous therapies. There are a number of malignancies that meet this requirement and for which we use extremely toxic drugs, as you are all aware.

However, it is important to remember that, although we as scientists know that certainty is unattainable, the American people, to a large degree, believe that uncertainty is unacceptable. It is also true that the American people have become very concerned about their personal health and are averse to risk taking. Thus, no FDA official has ever received a Medal of Honor for approval of a new drug! Indeed, I have never been able to find a person outside of the FDA, even among Smith, Kline & French people, who knows the name of the medical review officer primarily responsible for the approval of the breakthrough drug cimetidine (Tagamet).

In any case, it is indeed a slow and expensive process. Clearly, one must first identify a candidate drug. This is the primary concern, for example, of SeaPharm, as described in a later section. I suspect that those of you from that group would agree with me that three years might well be a very optimistic estimate for the time involved in carrying out preclinical animal testing for toxicity, filing an IND and having it approved, and then completing the various phases of clinical testing described above. Often, long-term animal studies should also be done, particularly if a drug that must be used over long periods of time might be a carcinogen or demonstrate chronic toxicity; this is usually done in parallel with the clinical testing, however, and need not delay the final approval. After completion of the NDA, a drug must undergo appropriate comparison by the FDA with other NDAs from competitors. The Agency does attempt to give preferential treatment to new molecular entities and to drugs that have potential in therapeutic areas in which only minimally effective drugs exist. Cimetidine, for example, was approved quite rapidly, and I hope that marine-derived drugs might meet the criteria for speedy processing. Such studies can easily take 10 to 20 years and require many millions of dollars; I suspect that today $30-50 million is a realistic figure.

The average time to approval does, of course, vary from country to country depending upon regulatory requirements, and the fact that the U.S. system results in the greatest time to approval in most cases has led to coining of the term "drug lag" for the time between approval in countries in western Europe such as the United Kingdom and approval in the United States. Unfortunately, it is difficult to make such comparisons in a meaningful fashion since application for registration is seldom made at the same time in more than one country and the requirements vary so widely, etc. However, there is no quarrel with the proposition that it usually takes longer in the United States. The question as to whether that is appropriate is a philosophic one that has long been argued by many people. I believe that delay is worthwhile, although I would like to see the process speeded up considerably; a discussion of this matter is, however, not part of today's presentation.

It is also worth noting that the Agency can and does give special consideration to drugs being developed for relatively rare diseases where the potential market is so small that it is not economically feasible to expend the sort of resources necessary to do a full NDA-type study. These so-called "orphan drugs" have been given special consideration, including financial support for their development, but nonetheless they must be demonstrated to meet the statutory safety and efficacy requirements of the Act.

Chief executive officers of some of the smaller high technology firms have often alleged that large manufacturers have told them that they could not possibly be successful in getting through the "FDA maze". It is important to understand that the FDA has a vested interest in encouraging the development of new useful drugs, and it is possible to get significant assistance from the FDA if you involve them in your thinking at an early stage in the development of a new drug. The recent approval of Human Growth Hormone for Genentech is an example of a small company's successfully obtaining approval of a new drug.

In closing, I would like to stress that, although the American public is not willing to accept it, Ralph Waldo Emerson was correct when he said, "Nature never gives anyone anything; it is always sold. It is only in the abstraction of ideals that choice comes without consequences". The responsibility of the FDA is to minimize the consequences by setting the "hurdles" at the proper height, but consequences there will be.

Section III

Current Research on Bioactive Compounds from Marine Sources

Isao Kitagawa
Faculty of Pharmaceutical Sciences, Osaka University, 1–6, Yamada-oka, Suita, Osaka 565, Japan

Studies in Marine Pharmaceutical Chemistry Research in Japanese Universities

INTRODUCTION

Marine life comprises many more species than does terrestrial life, so that one can expect to find a variety of chemically interesting marine-derived metabolites which are also bioactive. In recent years many marine natural products have been evaluated pharmacologically. Since these substances are chemically diverse, much attention has also been paid to their chemistry.

Marine metabolites thus far elucidated may be classified as: (1) bioactive substances, including (a) antimicrobial agents, (b) physiologically active substances (chemical signals) such as pheromones and allelochemics (allomones and kairomones), (c) pharmacologically active substances, and (d) cytotoxic and antitumor substances; (2) marine toxins; and (3) biochemical resources that may be converted to more valuable materials.

In this article I would like to describe marine pharmaceutical studies undertaken Japanese universities and then summarize our own work.

STUDIES ON MARINE NATURAL PRODUCTS IN JAPANESE UNIVERSITIES

In Japanese universities today, many scientists are engaged in chemical studies on marine metabolites. Their major interests may be ordered according to the subjects and methods of their recent investigations, as shown below:

A. Groups working mainly on physiologically active substances are guided by Professors T. Goto of Nagoya University (bioluminescence), S. Ikegami of Hiroshima University (echinoderm hormone), K. Ina of Shizuoka University (antifouling substances), T. Kajiwara of Yamaguchi University (algal gamete-attracting substances), H. Kamiya (invertebrate bioactive biopolymer) and H. Kawauchi of Kitasato University (fish hormonal protein and peptide), and T. Nomura of Tohoku University (physiologically active substances).

B. Groups working mainly on pharmacologically active substances are guided by Professors M. Fujiwara of Kyoto University (coral cardiotonic substances), N. Fusetani of the University of Tokyo (cell-division inhibiting substances), T. Higa of the University of the Ryukyus (environmental analysis), I. Kitagawa (bioactive substances) and T. Shiba (algal amino acid and peptide) of Osaka University, D. Uemura of Shizuoka University (antitumor polyether macrolide), and Y. Yamada of Tokyo College of Pharmacy (bioactive substances).

C. Marine toxins are being investigated by groups established by Professors K. Hashimoto of the University of Tokyo (phytoplankton toxins), Y. Hirata of Meijo University (marine toxins), T. Kosuge of Shizuoka College of Pharmacy (shellfish poisons), T. Okaichi of Kagawa University (phytoplankton toxins), and T. Yasumoto of Tohoku University (phytoplankton toxins).

D. Groups mainly engaged in studies of marine natural products from chemical and/or phytochemical viewpoints are those of Professors N. Ikekawa of Tokyo Institute of Technology (sterols), H. Kakisawa of Tsukuba University (algal metabolites), A. Kanazawa (sterols) and T. Katayama (carotenoids) of Kagoshima University, T. Kikuchi of Toyama Medical and Pharmaceutical University (algal metabolites), T. Komori of Kyushu University (asteroid metabolites), E. Kurosawa, T. Matsumoto, and T. Masamune of Hokkaido University (algal metabolites), M. Nakayama of Hiroshima University (marine metabolites), and T. Tokoroyama of Osaka City University (algal terpenoids).

RECENT MARINE PHARMACEUTICAL STUDIES

Of the many marine pharmaceutical studies reported recently by Japanese university scientists a few selected examples are:

Fusetani and his group isolated two novel nucleosides, mycalisines A (1) and B (2), from a marine sponge, *Mycale* sp. They have a cyano group and an anhydroribose moiety, and were discovered during monitoring of inhibition of cell division in fertilized starfish eggs.[1]

Fujiwara and his group found a remarkably cardiotonic peptide, Goniopora toxin (GPT) (3), in a stony coral *Goniopora* sp. The primary structure of GPT was determined as comprising 88 amino acids, and there was no primary structure similarity between GPT and other peptides such as the scorpion and sea anemone toxins. With regards to the mechanism of cardiotonic activity, it has been concluded that GPT defines a new locus on the extracellular aspect of the sodium channel that can selectively alter the process of inactivation.[2]

From the red alga *Laurencia obtusa*, Kurosawa and his group isolated two new cyclic polyethers with a squalene skeleton. One of them, teurilene (4), was characterized as having a *meso* structure, while the other, thyrsiferyl 23-acetate (5), was remarkably cytotoxic against P388 cells (ED_{50} 0.3 ng/ml).[3]

Hirata, Uemura, and their groups found several antitumor polyether macrolides from the marine sponge *Halichondria okadai*. Among them, halichondrin B (6) exhibited remarkable antitumor activity (IC_{50} 0.093 ng/ml; 2.5 μg/kg, T/C 203%) *vs*. B-16 melanoma, whereas norhalichondrin A (7) showed strong cytotoxicity (IC_{50} 5.2 ng/ml) *vs*. B-16 melanoma.[4]

During studies on diarrhetic shellfish poisoning, Yasumoto and his group identified four polyethers, the dinophysistoxins (8, 9) and the pectenotoxins (10, 11) from the dinoflagellates *Dinophysis forti* and *D. acuminata*.[5]

STUDIES AT OSAKA UNIVERSITY, FACULTY OF PHARMACEUTICAL SCIENCES

One of our major research subjects has been the chemical elucidation of bioactive marine natural products. I would like to summarize here our recent studies.

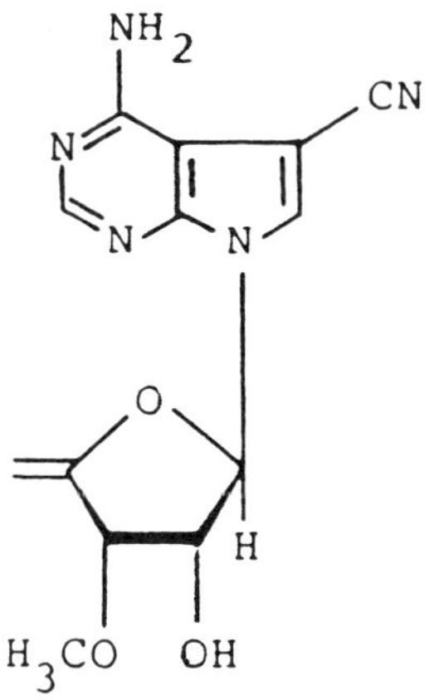

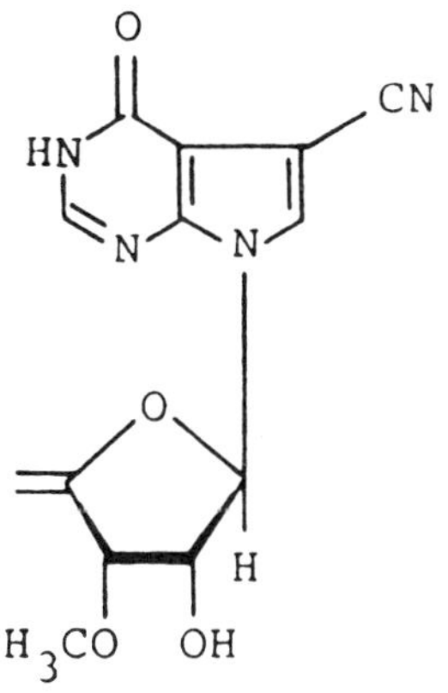

mycalisine A (1) mycalisine B (2)

```
1   5      10     15     20
PRGQI FGSCT CAWDE SEYPD
    25     30     35     40
KHGHS YGCGK KGHCW GQCRG
    45     50     55     60
LLSCG GAKEW CWIAE KHGDS
    65     70     75     80
DWLTC SKHSD CAVGI DNSNY
    85
MCWGS CSL
```

Goniopora toxin (3)

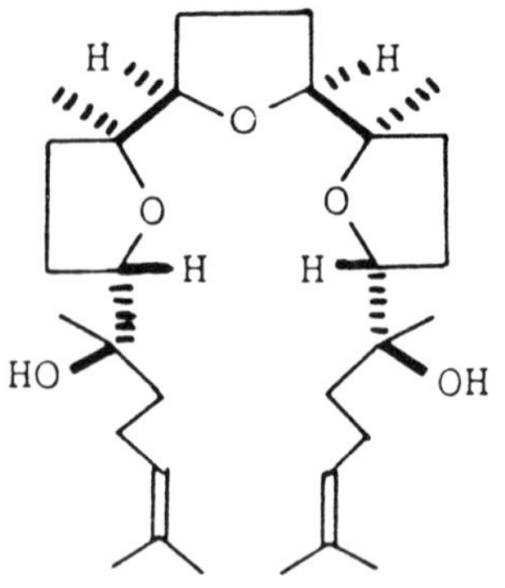

teurilene (4)

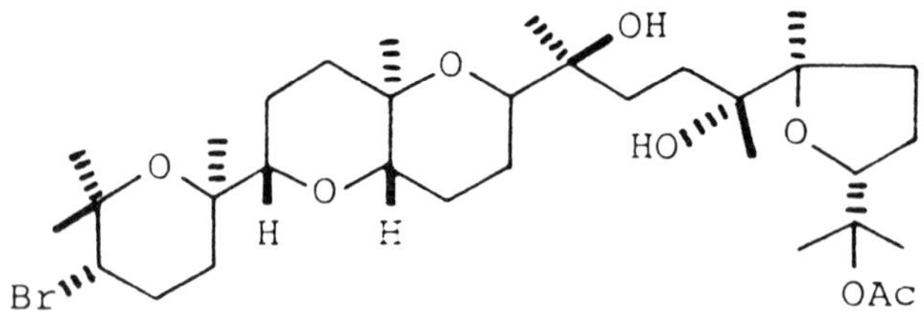

thyrsiferyl 23-acetate (5)

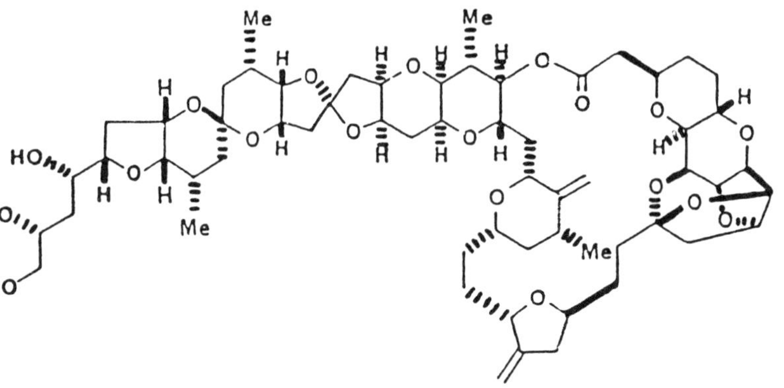

halichondrin B (6)

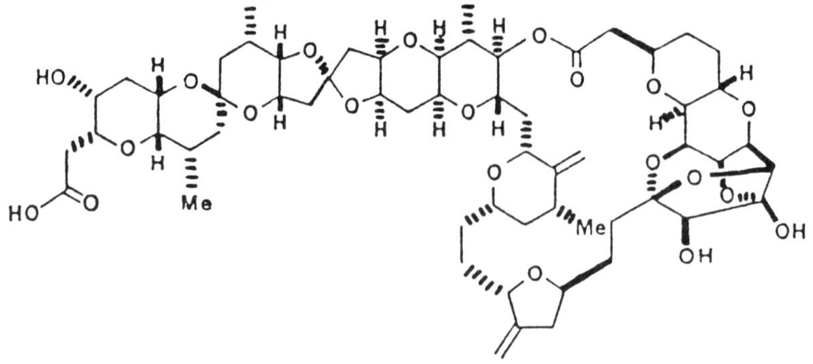

norhalichondrin A (7)

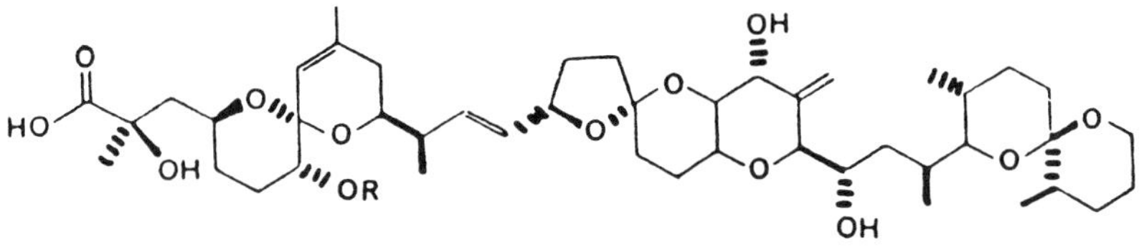

dinophysistoxin-1 : R = H (8)
dinophysistoxin-3 : R = acyl (9)

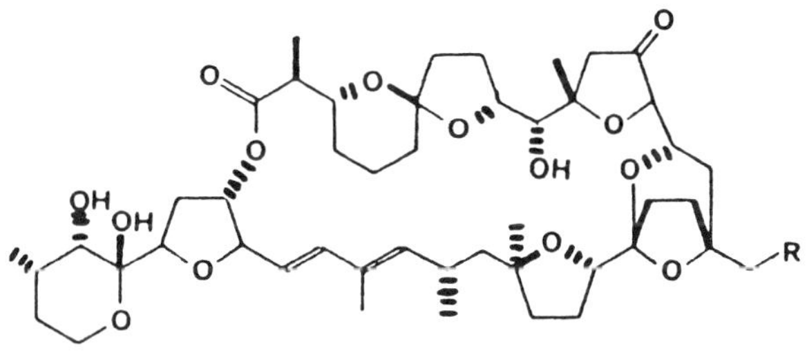

pectenotoxin-1 : R= OH (10)
pectenotoxin-2 : R= H (11)

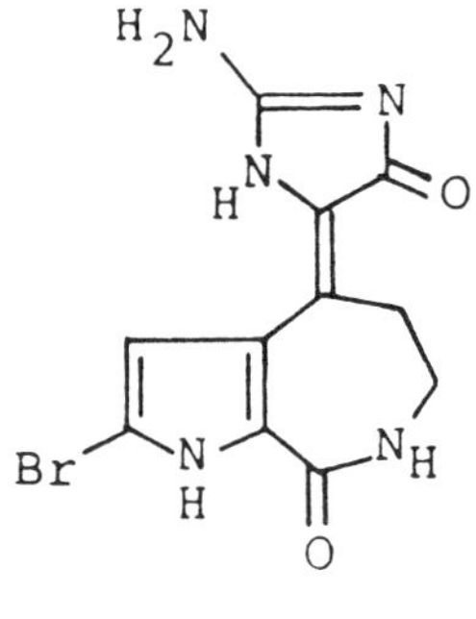

hymenialdisine (12)

A. Metabolites of Okinawan Marine Sponges. We have been investigating the constituents of marine sponges collected at Ishigaki-jima, Kohama-jima, and Zamami-jima Islands in Okinawa Prefecture (the southern islands of Japan). During these studies, we isolated various 3β-hydroxymethyl-A-nor-5α-cholestane derivatives and yellow pyrrole-containing guanidino pigments (*e.g.* hymenialdisine (12) from *Hymeniacidon aldis*,[6] and found several bioactive constituents from other marine sponges.

1. *Phyllospongia foliascens*. With monitoring of biological activities, the extract of the marine sponge was fractionated to give a galactolipid (M-5) (13)[7] and a bishomosesterterpene foliaspongin (16)[8] as the antiinflammatory principles. A sulfonoglucolipid (M-6) (14)[7] that inhibited a complement-fixation reaction was isolated from the same sponge. The structure of M-6 is closely related to that of another sulfonoglucolipid (ANT-1) (15), previously elucidated by us from the sea urchin *Anthocidaris crassispina*,[9] which did not inhibit the complement-fixation reaction. Foliaspongin is a 3-hydroxypentanoic acid ester of a bishomosesterterpene aldehyde. Recently, we re-investigated the lipophilic fraction of the same sponge and isolated several foliaspongin analogues. Among them, PF-9 (17) has been found to exhibit cytotoxic, antithrombocyte, and vasodilative activities.[10]

2. *Xestospongia sapra*. An inotropic constituent, halenaquinol (18) (ED_{50} 6 x 10^{-7} M against guinea pig left atria) and its monosulfate, halenaquinol sulfate (19), were isolated. Halenaquinol was photo-sensitive, thermolabile and readily oxidized to afford its quinonic counterpart, halenaquinone. The absolute stereochemistry of halenaquinol was determined by the application of the ^{13}C NMR LPSD method and by comparison of CD data for various derivatives with calculated CD values.[11,12] The mechanism of cardiotonic activity of halenaquinol is presumed to involve inhibition of cyclic AMP phosphodiesterase.[10]

B. Metabolites of Okinawan Soft Corals. The constituents of soft corals collected at Kohama-jima, Taketomi-jima, Iriomote-jima, and Zamami-jima Islands in Okinawa Prefecture have been investigated. In addition to chemically interesting substances--*ent*-valerenane sesquiterpenes [valerenenol (20), isovalerenenol (21), anhydrovalerenenol (22)] from *Xenia* sp.;[13] a diterpene having a novel skeleton, alcyonolide (23), from *Alcyonium* sp.;[14] a pair of perhydroazulene diterpene diastereomers, xeniolone (24) and isoxeniolone (25), from *Xenia* sp.[15]--the following bioactive substances were identified.

1. *Alcyonium* sp. Five pregnane glycosides of moderate antibiotic activity were isolated. The structure of these glycosides, pregnediosides-a (26) and -b (29), and their monoacetates (27, 28, 30) were determined by a partial synthesis of their common aglycone, 3β,4α-dihydroxy-5α-pregn-20-ene, and by physical data analyses.[16] Although pregn-20-ene steroids were reported from several soft corals and a gorgonian, these steroids have not been isolated previously in glyco-conjugated forms. Except for echinoderm saponins, pregnediosides were the first steroidal glycosides isolated from marine organisms.

2. *Clavularia koellikeri*. Three new trinorsesquiterpenes, clavukerins A (31),[17] B (32), and C (33),[18] were isolated from this stolonifer. Among these, clavukerin C was characterized as possessing a hydroperoxy function, rare in nature. The composition of these chemical constituents in the stolonifer was found to vary with the year of collection, although each stolonifer was collected in the same area during the same season. From the stolonifer collected in 1983 we found, in addition to the above-mentioned trinorsesquiterpenes, a new diterpene having a methyl-migrated dolabellane skeleton, neodolabelline (34).[19]

Endo and his group previously isolated two cytotoxic substances, clavularins A (35) and B (36),[20] from *C. koellikeri*. However, we have been unable, so far, to detect these compounds, and we presume that clavularin B might be a secondary product formed from

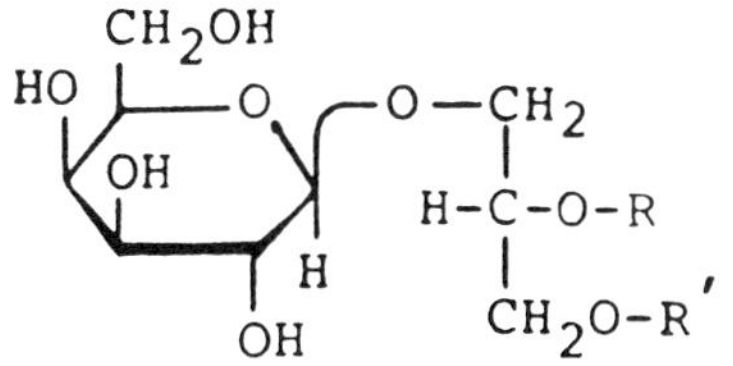

M-5 (13)

a:b:c = 1:10:10

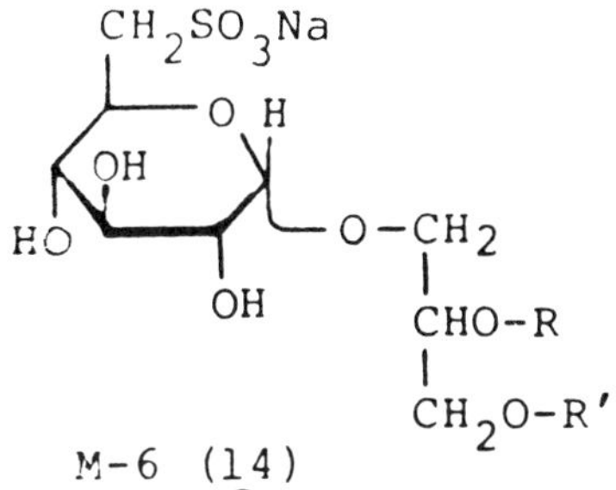

M-6 (14)

b:c = 1:2

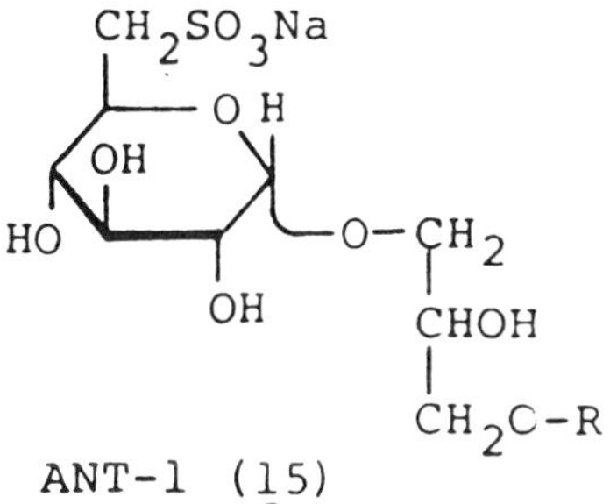

ANT-1 (15)

a:c = 1:24

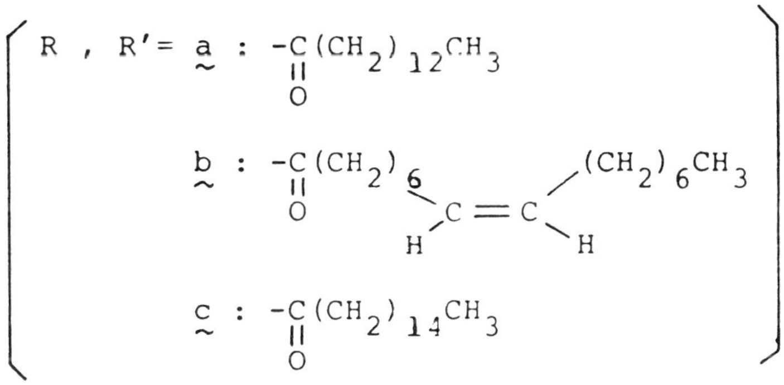

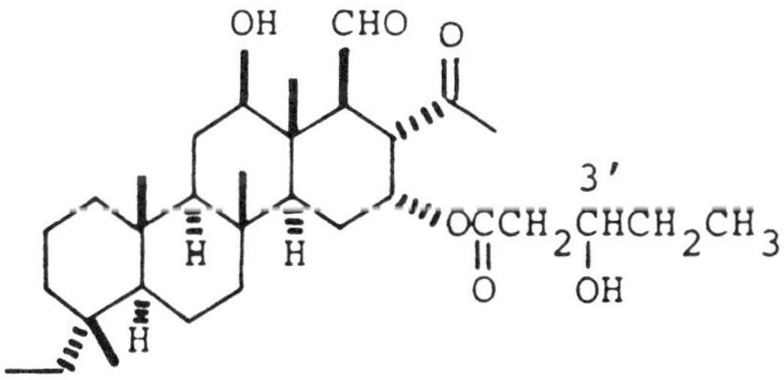

foliaspongin (16)

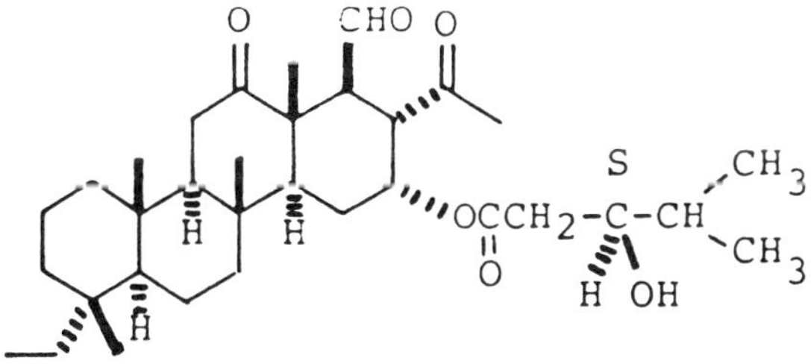

PF-9 (17)

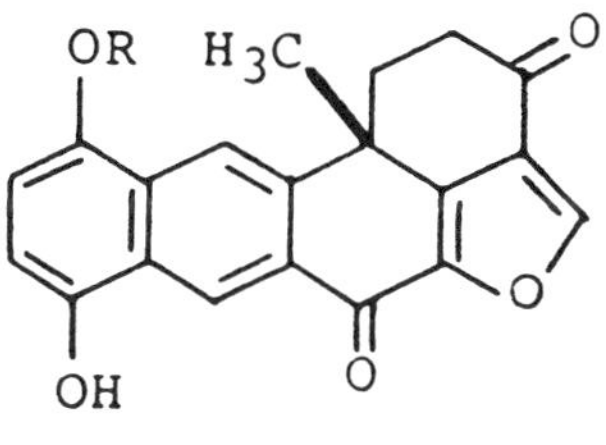

halenaquinol (18)
$R = H$

halenaquinol sulfate (19)
$R = SO_3Na$

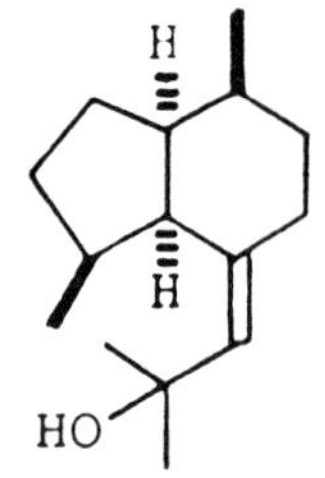

valerenenol (20)

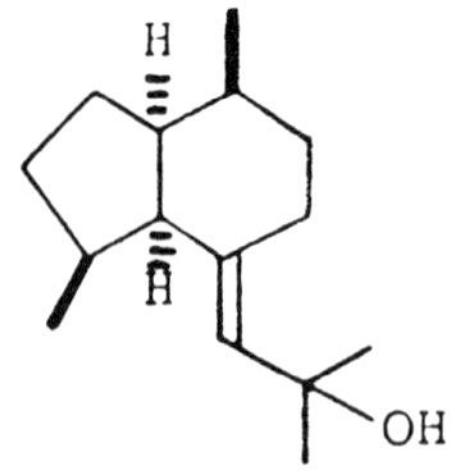

isovalerenenol (21)

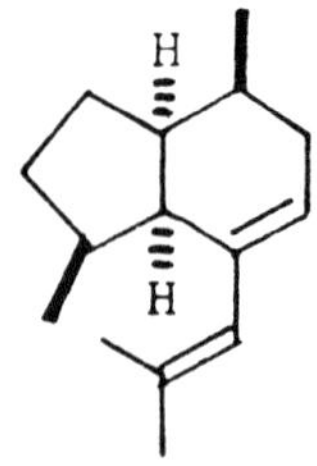

anhydro-valerenenol (22)

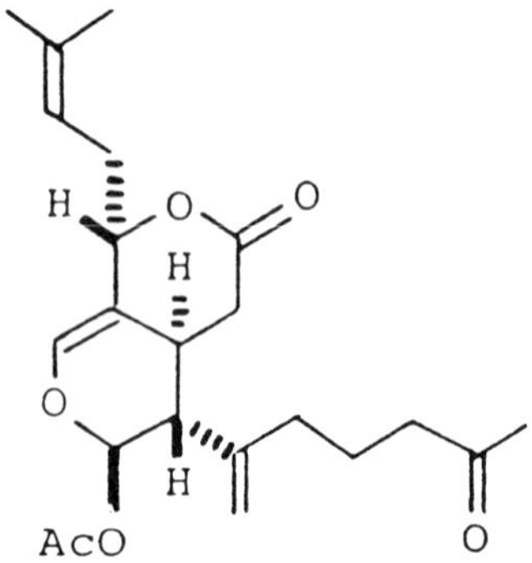

alcyonolide (23)

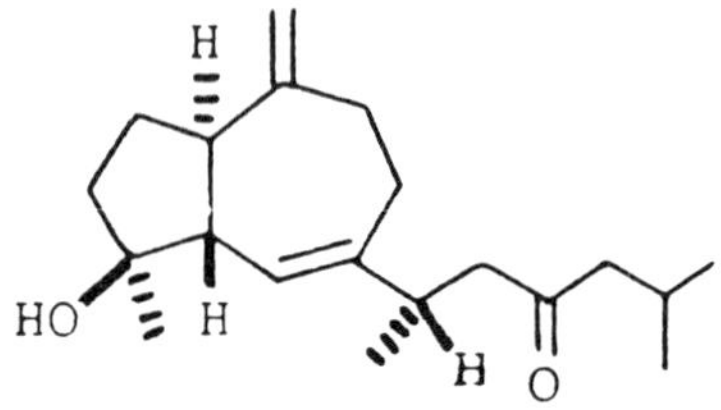

xeniolone (24)

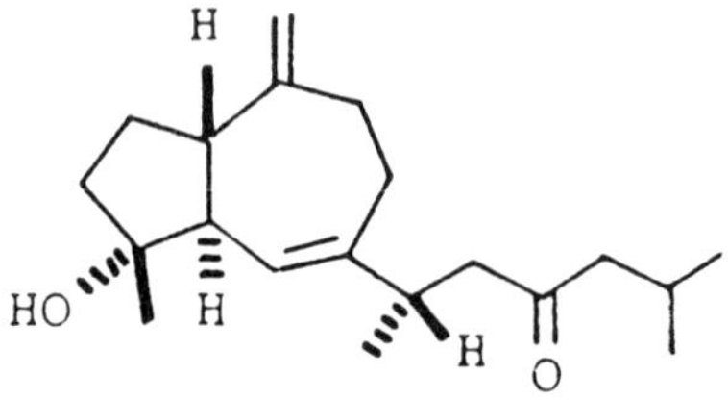

isoxeniolone (25)

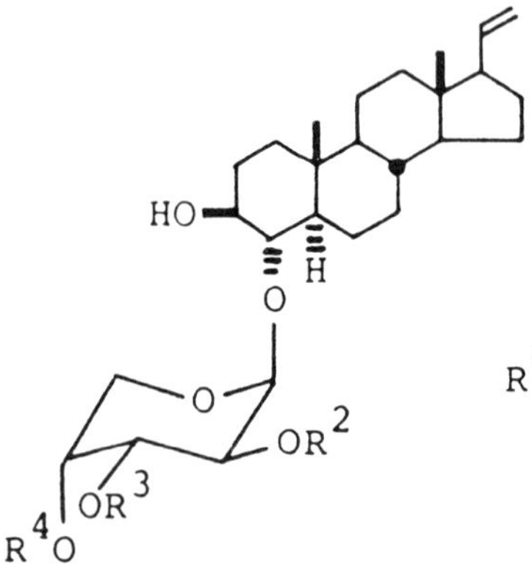

26 : $R^2=R^3=R^4=H$

(pregnedioside-a)

27 : $R^2=R^4=H$, $R^3=Ac$

28 : $R^2=R^3=H$, $R^4=Ac$

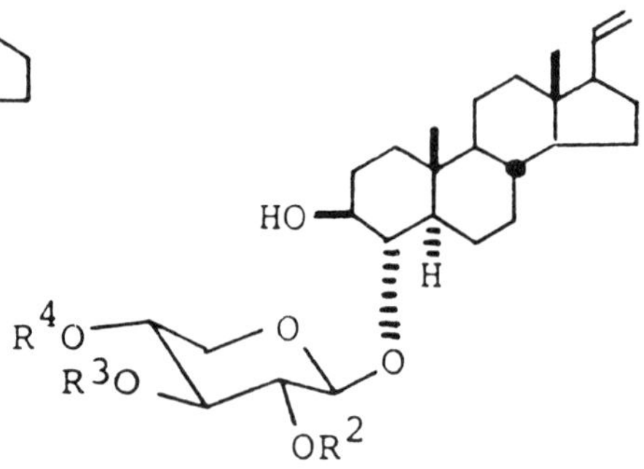

29 : $R^2=R^3=R^4=H$

(pregnedioside-b)

30 : $R^2=R^3=H$, $R^4=Ac$

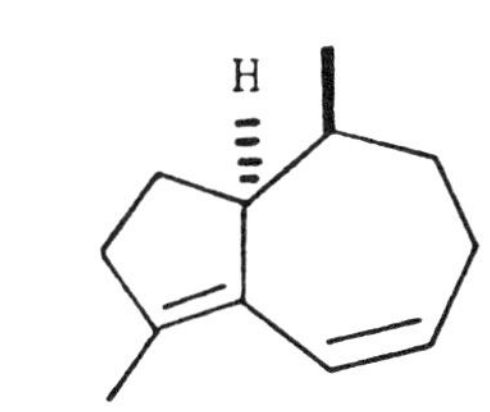

clavukerin A (31)

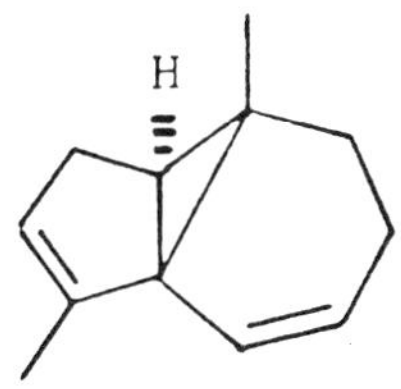

clavukerin B (32)

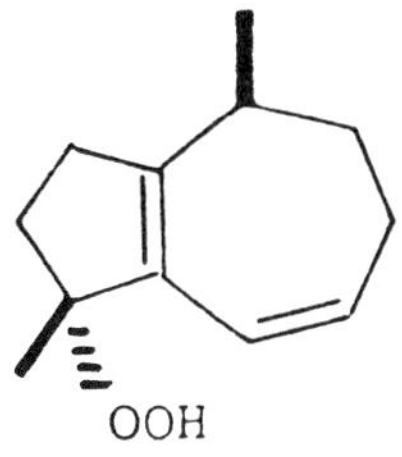

clavukerin C (33)

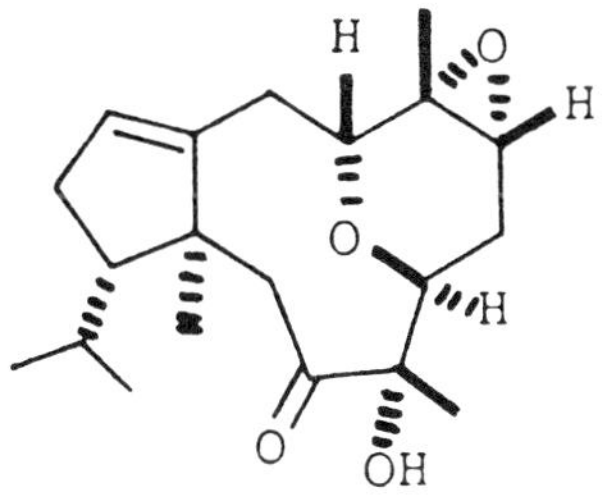

neodolabelline (34)

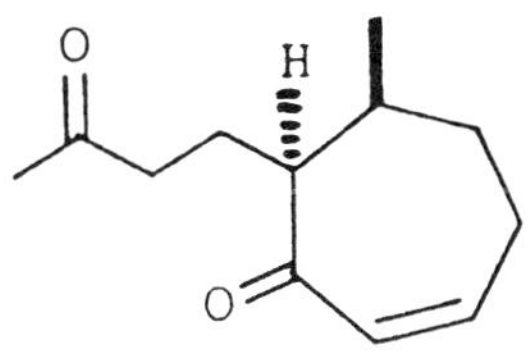

clavularin A (35)

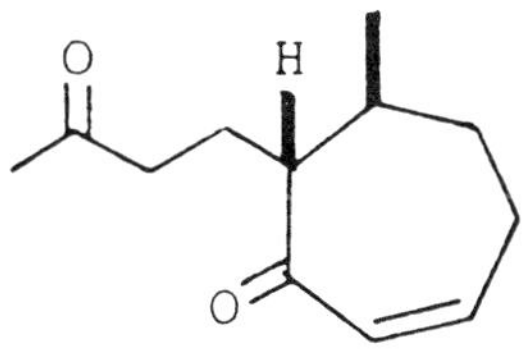

clavularin B (36)

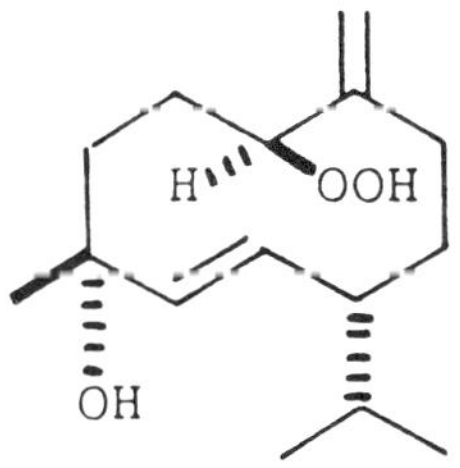

nephtheoxydiol (37)

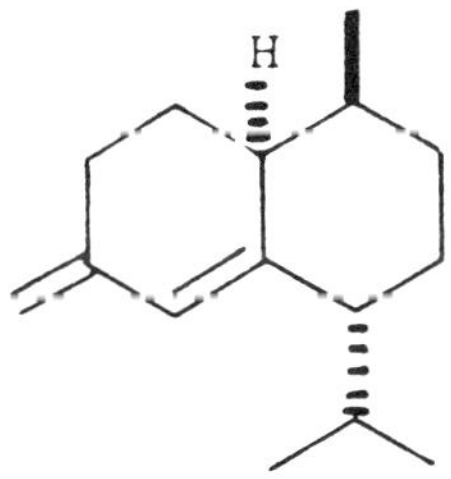

nephthene (38)

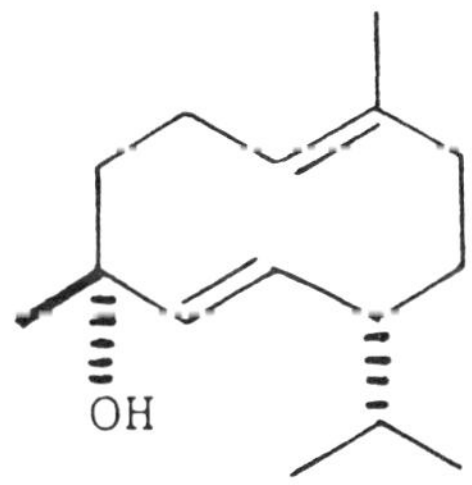

nephthenol (39)

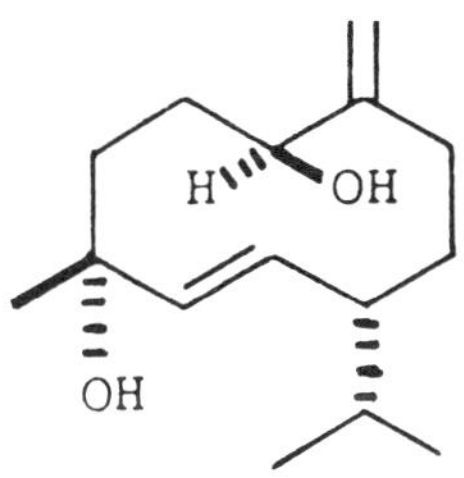

nephthediol (40)

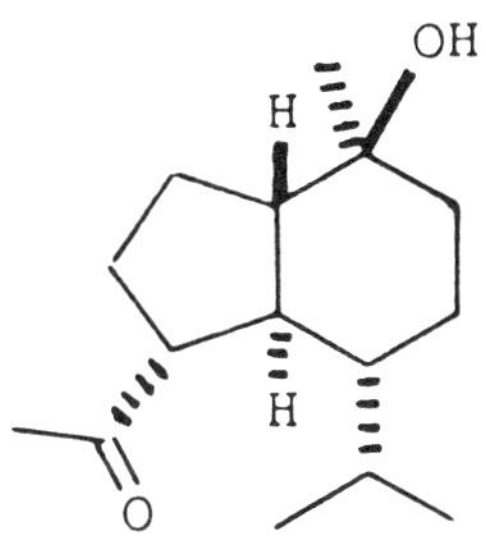

ent-oplopanone (41)

the unstable clavukerin C during the isolation procedure. Clavukerin B was recently isolated by Fenical and his group from the Palau stolonifer *C. inflata* var. *luzoniana* as an ichthyotoxic principle.[21]

3. *Nephthea* sp. From this soft coral, we recently isolated a new hydroperoxy sesquiterpene, nephtheoxydiol (37), together with four new, related sesquiterpenes (38-41).[10] As was shown in the quantitative photosensitized oxidative conversion of clavukerin A to clavukerin C, photooxidation of nephthenol (39) has provided quantitatively nephtheoxydiol, a comparatively stable compound. Nephtheoxydiol has been found to exhibit cytotoxic activity (IC_{50} 0.1 μg/ml *vs.* B-16 melanoma).[10]

4. *Clavularia viridis.* Early in our chemical studies we isolated new *ent*-prostanoids (the name eicosanoid has been proposed recently), claviridenones-a (42), -b (43), -c (44), and -d (45), and 20-acetoxyclaviridenones-b (46) and -c (47), which were characterized by a cross-conjugated 5,7-dien-9-on-10-ene chromophore.[22] The claviridenones are geometrical isomers at their 5,7-diene moieties and are interconverted by irradiation with fluorescent lamps. Claviridenones were found to exhibit significant cytotoxicity (IC_{50} 0.2-0.4 μg/ml for L1210) and antitumor activity (P388 and Ehrlich ascites). Further investigation of the same stolonifer yielded four new antitumor steroids (1-T/C 69% at 1 μg/ml *vs.* P388): stoloniferones-a (48), -b (49), -c (50), and -d (51).[23] Stoloniferones differ from each other only in their side chains and possess a common steroidal skeleton with oxygen functions similar to those often found in Solanaceous antitumor steroids.

It has been suggested that the bioactive compounds hitherto isolated from marine sponges and soft corals are not endogenous but are biosynthesized by photosynthetic unicellular algal symbionts. In order to clarify this matter for claviridenones and stoloniferones, we recently isolated the algal symbiont of *C. viridis*, and by HPLC, analyzed the distribution of these bioactive constituents in the symbiont and in several parts of the stolonifer. So far we have found that claviridenones are biosynthesized mainly by the algal symbiont, while stoloniferones are produced endogenously by the stolonifer.[10]

C. Echinoderm Saponins. The phylum Echinodermata comprises five classes: Asteroidea (starfish), Crinoidea (sea lily), Echinoidea (sea urchin), Holothuroidea (sea cucumber), and Ophiuroidea (brittle star). Among these, Asteroidea and Holothuroidea are unique in the animal kingdom, since they include various species which metabolize steroidal and triterpenoidal oligoglycosides (saponins) which function as allomones (also as kairomones in some Asteroidea). In the course of our continuing studies of oligoglycosides of botanical origin, we have investigated the oligoglycosidic constituents of the starfish "crown of thorns", *Acanthaster planci*, and of 19 species of sea cucumber.

Starfish are carnivorous and metabolize steroidal oligoglycosides which function as both allomones and kairomones. The starfish *Acanthaster planci* is the natural enemy of corals; some years ago this starfish posed a considerable threat to coral reefs in the Okinawa Prefecture of Japan. We isolated the major toxic, saponin thornasteroside A (52) from the starfish and elucidated its structure.[24]

Our investigation of oligoglycosidic constituents of sea cucumbers started with *Stichopus japonicus*, whose constituents were reported to exhibit significant antifungal activity. After completion of this work in 1978, we conducted chemical analyses of the oligoglycosidic constituents of other sea cucumbers collected mostly in Okinawa Prefecture.

1. Triterpenoidal Oligoglycosides without a Sulfate Group. **Holotoxins A (53) and B (54)** were isolated from the whole body of the sea cucumber *Stichopus japonicus* and were found to exhibit significant growth-inhibitory activity against pathogenic microorganisms such as *Trichophyton, Candida, Trichomonas, Aspergillus* and *Penicillium* spp.[25] They were hexaglycosides of holotoxigenol, a lanostane sapogenol having a 16-keto-

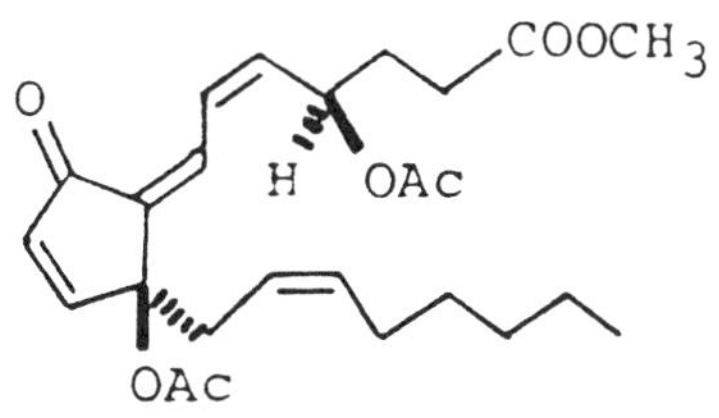

claviridenone-a (42)

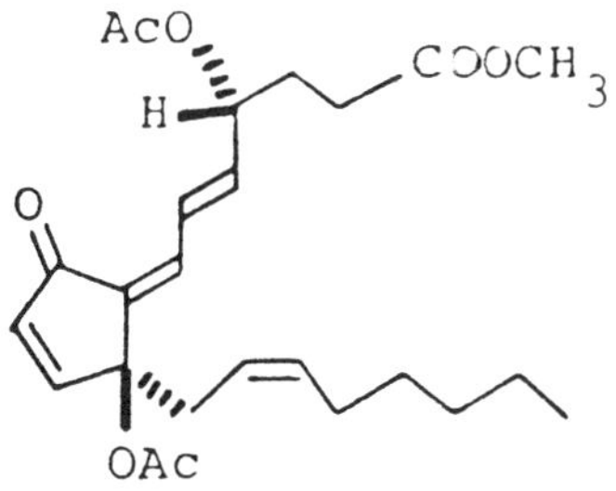

claviridenone-b (43)

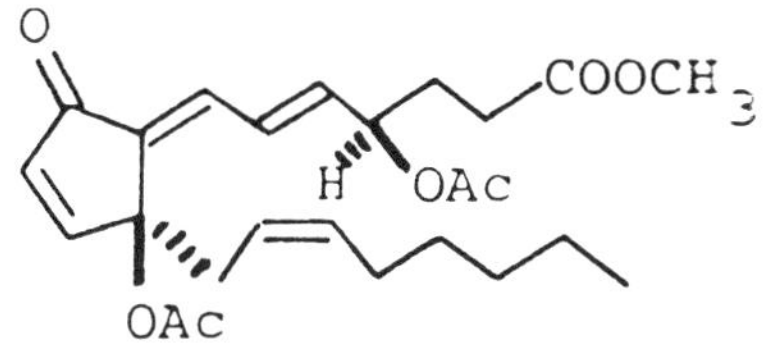

claviridenone-c (44)

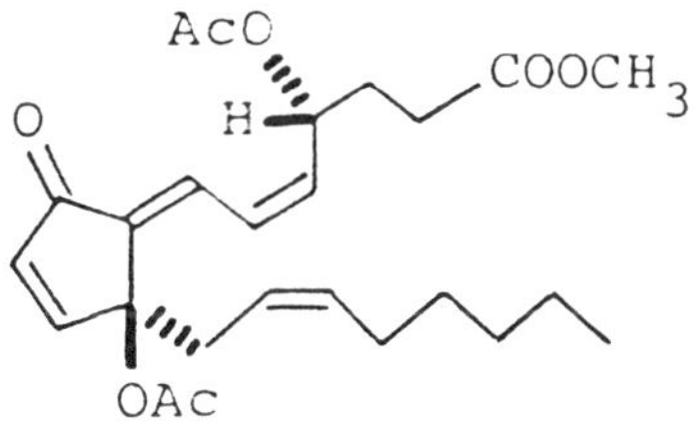

claviridenone-d (45)

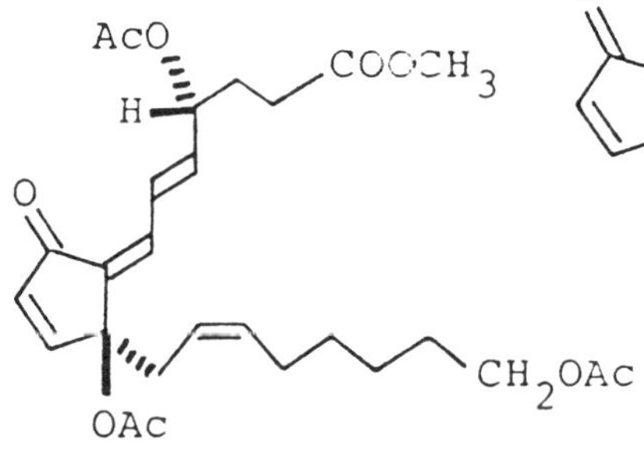

20-acetoxy-claviridenone-b (46)

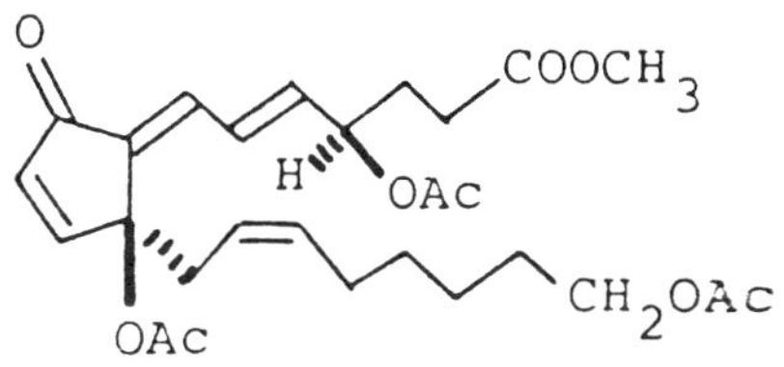

20-acetoxy-claviridenone-c (47)

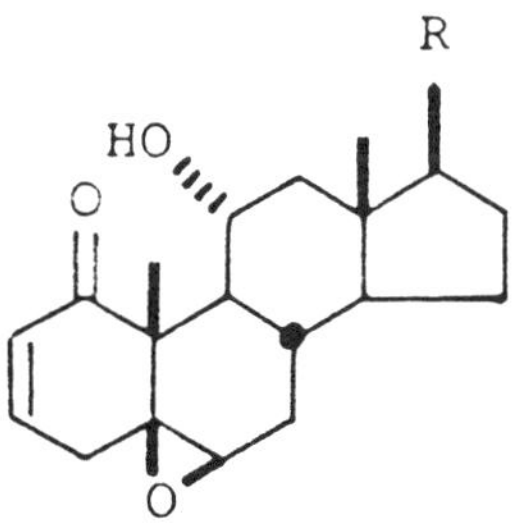

R = 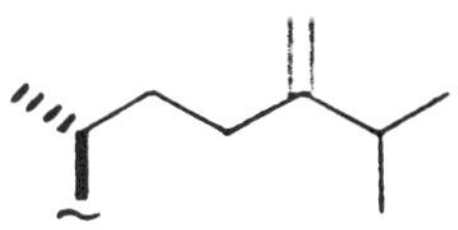 stoloniferone-a (48)

R = 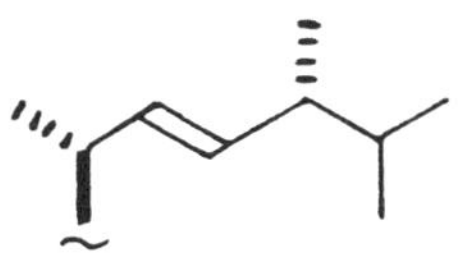 stoloniferone-b (49)

R = 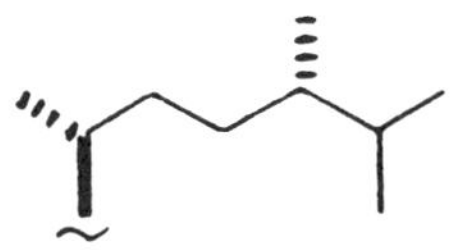 stoloniferone-c (50)

R = 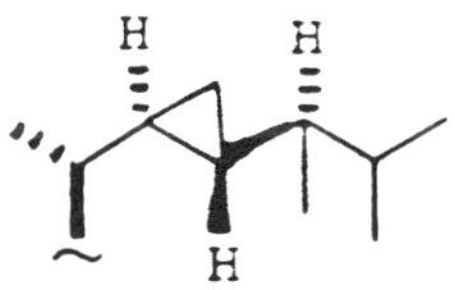 stoloniferone-d (51)

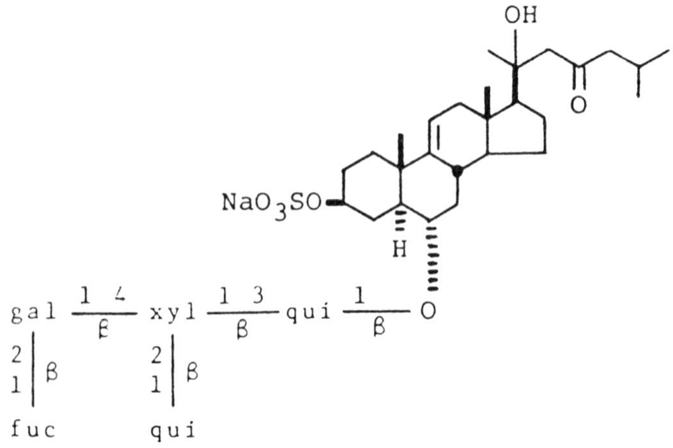

thornasteroside A (52)

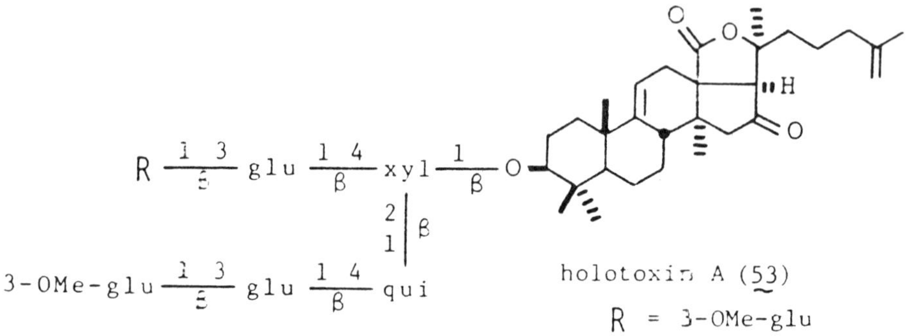

holotoxin A (53)
R = 3-OMe-glu

holotoxin B (54)
R = glu

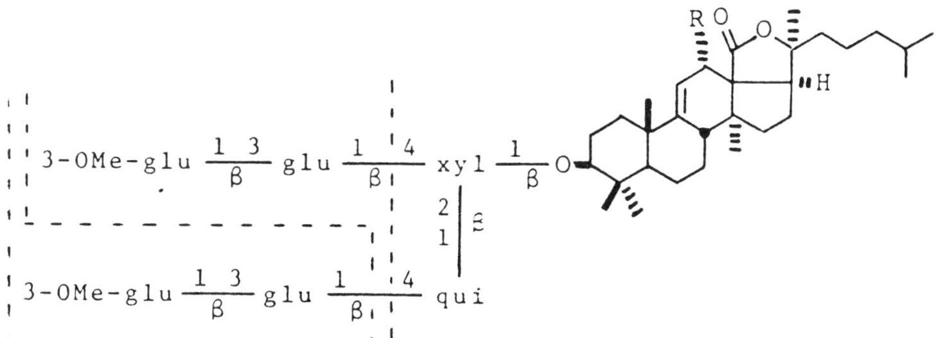

bivittoside A (55) R = OH

bivittoside B (56) R = OH

bivittoside C (57) R = H

bivittoside D (58) R = OH

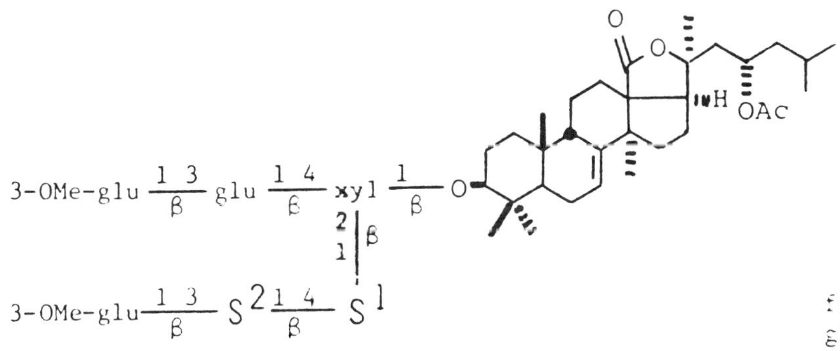

stichloroside A_1 (59) S^1= xyl , S^2= glu

A_2 (60) S^1= xyl , S^2= glu , Δ^{25}

stichloroside B_1 (61) S^1= glu , S^2= xyl

B_2 (62) S^1= glu , S^2= xyl , Δ^{25}

stichloroside C_1 (63) S^1= qui , S^2= xyl

C_2 (64) S^1= qui , S^2= xyl , Δ^{25}

fuc= fucose
glu= glucose
3-OMe-glu= 3-OMe-glucose
gal= galactose
qui= quinovose
xyl= xylose

18,20-γ-lactone moiety. Holotoxins were the key compounds in our subsequent search for antifungal constituents in various sea cucumbers.

Bivittosides A (55), B (56), C (57), and D (58), four new triterpenoidal oligoglycosides, were isolated from the Cuvierian tubules and the body wall of the sea cucumber *Bohadschia bivittata*. Bivittosides A, B, and D were, respectively, di-, tetra-, and hexa-glycosides of a common lanostane sapogenol having a 12α-hydroxy-18,20-γ-lactone moiety, while bivittoside C was the hexaglycoside lacking the 12α-hydroxy group.[26]

Stichlorosides A_1 (59), A_2 (60), B_1 (61), B_2 (62), C_1 (63), and C_2 (64), six new sapogenol hexaglycosides, were isolated from the body wall of the sea cucumber *Stichopus chloronotus*.[27] All six stichlorosides possessed a $\Delta^{7(8)}$ double bond that is characteristic of these sea cucumber saponins; among those structures hitherto elucidated in our laboratory most have a $\Delta^{9(11)}$ double bond in their sapogenol parts.

2. Triterpenoidal Oligoglycosides with a Sulfate Group. **Holothurins A (67)**[28] **and B (65)**[29] were isolated from the body wall and the Cuvierian tubules of the sea cucumber *Holothuria leucospilota*. Holothurin B exhibited acute toxicity (LD_{50} 14.9 mg/kg, i.p., mice) and affected skeletal muscle (frog) and smooth muscle (guinea pig) contractions. Holothurin A was later isolated from several other sea cucumbers--*Holothuria atra, H. edulis, H. axiologa, Actinopyga agassizi*, and *Bohadschia graeffei*--whereas holothurin B was found only in *H. atra*.[10]

Echinosides A (71) and B (68) were isolated[30] from the body wall of the sea cucumber *Actinopyga echinites*. Each echinoside contained a sulfate group attached to its xylosyl unit and their carbohydrate sequences were identical with those in holothurins A and B, respectively. Later, echinoside A was isolated from *Holothuria atra, H. scabra, H. axiologa, A. mauritiana*, and *Bohadschia graeffei*, and echinoside B from *H. atra* and *A. mauritiana*.[10] It is interesting to note that the sea cucumber *B. graeffei* produces a large amount of echinoside A (*ca.* 0.9 g from the body wall of one animal).[10]

24-Dehydroechinosides A and B. In the 1960's, "holothurin A", isolated from the Cuvierian tubules of the Bahamian sea cucumber *Actinopyga agassizi*, received much attention because of its various biological activities (*e.g.*, LD_{50} 9 mg/kg, i.v., mice; piscicidal, hemolytic, and cytotoxic activity; and blockage of the neuromuscular synapse). In 1969, Chanley and his group proposed a partial structure for "holothurin A", but they could not isolate the oligoglycoside in pure form. Since a preserved sample of the Cuvierian tubules of *A. agassizi* became available to us by courtesy of Profs. Ciereszko and Schmitz of the University of Oklahoma, we analyzed the oligoglycosidic constituents and found that "holothurin A" was a 3:1 mixture of 24-dehydroechinoside A (72) and holothurin A.[31] Later, 24-dehydroechinosides A (72) and B (69) were also isolated from *A. mauritiana*.[10]

3. Antimicrobial Activities of Sea Cucumber Oligoglycosides. During our investigation of sea cucumber oligoglycosides, *ca.* 40 analogues with structural variations in their sapogenol and/or carbohydrate moieties became available. Since holotoxins A and B showed significant growth-inhibition against pathogenic microorganisms, we examined the antimicrobial activities of their analogues from the viewpoint of structure-activity relationship. So far, it is clear that the following structural features are essential for antifungal activity: (1) oxygen function(s) in the vicinity of the 18,20-γ-lactone moiety in the lanostane sapogenol, and (2) a linear sequence of monosaccharide constituents in the carbohydrate moiety, as seen in echinoside A (71), but without the sulfate group.

4. Pharmacological Activity of Sea Cucumber Oligoglycosides. Holothurin A, desulfated holothurin A (66), echinoside A, and desulfated echinoside A (70) effected prolonged contractions of excised rabbit aorta in a dose-response manner. These contractions were shown to be caused by the increase of Ca^{2+} permeability in the cell mem-

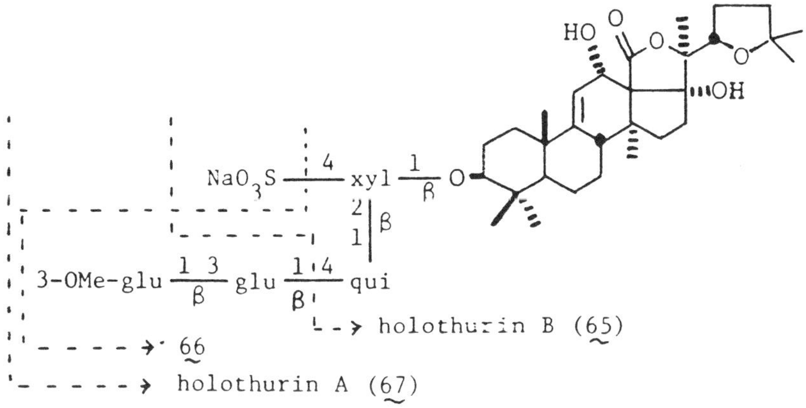
HO
O
O
OH
NaO3S
4
xyl
1
β
O
2
1
β
3-OMe-glu
1 3
β
glu
1 4
β
qui
holothurin B (65)
66
holothurin A (67)

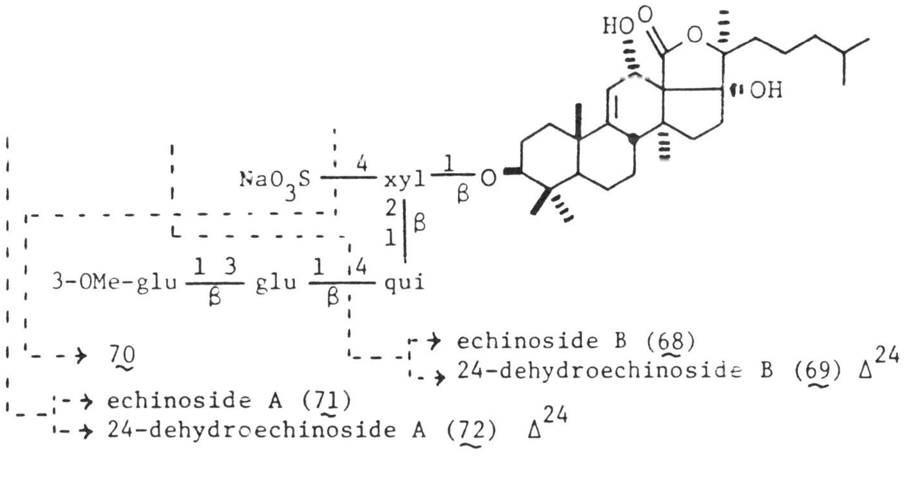
HO
O
O
OH
NaO3S
4
xyl
1
β
O
2
1
β
3-OMe-glu
1 3
β
glu
1 4
β
qui
echinoside B (68)
24-dehydroechinoside B (69) Δ24
70
echinoside A (71)
24-dehydroechinoside A (72) Δ24

brane of smooth muscle. Among sea cucumber saponins examined for their inhibiting activities against Na,K-ATPase, echinoside A was shown to be the most active (IC_{50} $2x10^{-5}$M). These oligoglycosides showed non-competitive inhibition of ATP and K^+.

REFERENCES

1. Kato, Y.; Fusetani, N.; Matsunaga, S.; Hashimoto, K.; *Tetrahedron Lett*, 1985, *26*, 3483.
2. Fujiwara, M. *et al.*, to be published.
3. Suzuki, T.; Suzuki, M.; Furusaki, A.; Matsumoto, T.; Kato, A.; Imanaka, Y.; Kurosawa, E., *Tetrahedron Lett.*, 1982, *26*, 1329.
4. Uemura, D.; Takahashi, K.; Yamamoto, T.; Katayama, C.; Tanaka, J.; Okumura, Y.; Hirata, Y., *J. Am. Chem. Soc.*, 1985, *107*, 4796.
5. Yasumoto, T.; Murata, M.; Oshima, Y.; Sano, M.; Matsumoto, G.K.; Clardy, J., *Tetrahedron*, 1985, *41*, 1019.
6. Kitagawa, I.; Kobayashi, M.; Kitanaka, K.; Kido, M.; Kyogoku, Y., *Chem. Pharm. Bull.*, 1983, *31*, 2321.
7. Kikuchi, H.; Tsukitani, Y.; Manda, T.; Fujii, T.; Nakanishi, M.; Kobayashi, M.; Kitagawa, I., *Chem. Pharm. Bull.*, 1982, *30*, 3544.
8. Kikuchi, H.; Tsukitani, Y.; Shimizu, I.; Kobayashi, M.; Kitagawa, I. *Chem. Pharm. Bull.*, 1983, *31*, 552.
9. Kitagawa, I.; Hamamoto, Y.; Kobayashi, M., *Chem. Pharm. Bull.*, 1979, *27*, 1934.
10. Kitagawa, I. *et al.*, to be published.
11. Kobayashi, M.; Shimizu, N.; Kyogoku, Y.; Kitagawa, I., *Chem. Pharm. Bull.*, 1985, *33*, 1305.
12. Kobayashi, M.; Shimizu, N.; Kitagawa, I.; Kyogoku, Y.; Harada, N.; Uda, H., *Tetrahedron Lett.*, 1985, *26*, 3833.
13. Kobayashi, M.; Yasuzawa, T.; Kyogoku, Y.; Kido, M.; Kitagawa, I., *Chem. Pharm. Bull.*, 1982, *30*, 3431.
14. Kobayashi, M.; Yasuzawa, T.; Kitagawa, I.; Kobayashi, Y.; Kyogoku, Y., *Tetrahedron Lett.*, 1981, *22*, 4445.
15. Kobayashi, M.; Cui, Z.; Cai, Y.; Kyogoku, Y.; Kitagawa, I., *Chem. Pharm. Bull.*, 1985, *33*, 1309.
16. Kobayashi, M.; Kiyota, Y.; Orito, S.; Kyogoku, Y.; Kitagawa, I., *Tetrahedron Lett.*, 1984, *25*, 3731.
17. Kobayashi, M.; Son, B.W.; Kido, M.; Kyogoku, Y.; Kitagawa, I., *Chem. Pharm. Bull.*, 1983, *31*, 2160.
18. Kobayashi, M.; Son, B.W.; Kyogoku, Y.; Kitagawa, I., *Chem. Pharm. Bull.*, 1984, *32*, 1667.
19. Kobayashi, M.; Son, B.W.; Fujiwara, T.; Kyogoku, Y.; Kitagawa, I., *Tetrahedron Lett.*, 1984, *25*, 5543.
20. Endo, M.; Nakagawa, M.; Hamamoto, Y.; Nakanishi, T., *J. Chem. Soc., Chem. Commun.*, 1983, 980.
21. Izac, R.R.; Fenical, W.; Wright, J.M., *Tetrahedron Lett.*, 1984, *25*, 1325.
22. Kitagawa, I.; Kobayashi, M.; Yasuzawa, T.; Son, B.W.; Yoshihara, M.; Kyogoku, Y., *Tetrahedron Lett.*, 1985, *41*, 995.
23. Kobayashi, M.; Lee, N.K.; Son, B.W.; Yanagi, K.; Kyogoku, Y.; Kitagawa, I., *Tetrahedron Lett.*, 1984, *25*, 5925.
24. Kitagawa, I.; Kobayashi, M., *Chem. Pharm. Bull.*, 1978, *26*, 1864.
25. Kitagawa, I.; Yamanaka, H.; Kobayashi, M.; Nishino, T.; Yosioka, I.; Sugawara, T., *Chem. Pharm. Bull.*, 1978, *26*, 3722.
26. Kitagawa, I.; Kobayashi, M.; Hori, M.; Kyogoku, Y., *Chem. Pharm. Bull.*, 1981, *29*, 282.

27. Kitagawa, I.; Kobayashi, M.; Inamoto, T.; Yasuzawa, T.; Kyogoku, Y., *Chem. Pharm. Bull.*, 1981, *29*, 2387.
28. Kitagawa, I.; Nishino, T.; Kobayashi, M.; Kyogoku, Y., *Chem. Pharm. Bull.*, 1981, *29*, 1951.
29. Kitagawa, I.; Nishino, T.; Kobayashi, M.; Matsuno, T.; Akutsu, H.; Kyogoku, Y., *Chem. Pharm. Bull.*, 1981, *29*, 1942.
30. Kitagawa, I.; Kobayashi, M.; Inamoto, T.; Fuchida, M.; Kyogoku, Y., *Chem. Pharm. Bull.*, 1985, *33*, 5214.
31. Kitagawa, I.; Kobayashi, M.; Kyogoku, Y., *Chem. Pharm. Bull.*, 1982, *30*, 2045.

Jun'ichi Kobayashi, Hideshi Nakamura, Yasushi Ohizumi, Masaki Kobayashi
Mitsubishi-Kasei Institute of Life Sciences, 11 Minamiooya, Machida-shi, Tokyo 194, Japan
Yoshimasa Hirata
Faculty of Pharmacy, Meijo University, Nagoya 468, Japan

Research on Marine Natural Products at the Mitsubishi-Kasei Institute of Life Sciences

In the field of marine natural products chemistry much attention has been paid recently to bioactive substances. Chemical studies of such substances are expected not only to reveal compounds with unique structures, but also to lead to the development of new medicines of value to mankind. We have been interested primarily in isolating and determining the structures of bioactive natural products from Okinawan marine sources. Assay systems using isolated mammalian muscle preparations (guinea pig atrium and ileum, rabbit aorta, etc.), enzymes (Na,K-ATPase, etc.), and microorganisms (bacteria, fungi, etc.) have been applied to 70% ethanol extracts of several hundred marine invertebrates (gastropods, sponges, soft corals, tunicates, etc.) collected in Okinawan waters.

Pharmacologically Active Substances from the Venoms of Cone Shells. Most species of the gastropod family Conidae possess a potent venom, which is used primarily to capture prey such as small fishes, other gastropods, or polychaete worms. The 400 species of cone shells in the tropical and subtropical seas of the world produce a variety of venoms, which differ according to the feeding habits of the producing animal. The venoms of fish-eating cone shells such as *Conus geographus*, *C. striatus*, and *C. magus* are lethal to fish and mice and dangerous even for humans, whereas those of shell-eating cones such as *C. textile* show little if any such activity.[1] The venoms of worm-eating cones such as *C. eburneus* and *C. tessulatus* are lethal to fish but not to mice.

By monitoring their effects on isolated mammalian muscle preparations, we have obtained the active principles of several cone shell venoms and have characterized their pharmacological properties. Two basic 22-residue peptide toxins, geographutoxins I (1) and II (2) from the venom of *C. geographus*,[2-4] inhibited the contractile response of the mouse diaphragm to direct stimulation, possibly by blocking sodium channels in the skeletal muscle cell membrane. In frog skeletal muscle, however, much higher concentrations of the toxins were required to suppress the contractile response. Geographutoxins I and II are unique examples of peptidic sodium channel blockers with a marked species-dependent specificity.

Striatoxin, a powerful cardiotonic glycoprotein (mol wt, 25,000), isolated from the venom of *C. striatus*,[6] produced a biphasic contraction of the guinea pig ileum[5] and a positive inotropic effect on the atrium. Two cardiotonic polypeptides (mol wt, *ca.* 45,000 and 1,500) from the venom of *C. magus* have been purified.[7,8] These three toxins caused a marked, long-lasting inotropic action, which may be caused by increased sodium ion permeability of the cardiac cell membrane.

5 10
Arg-Asp-Cys-Cys-Thr-Hyp-Hyp-Lys-Lys-Cys-Lys-Asp-Arg-Gln-
15 20
Cys-Lys-Hyp-Gln-Arg-Cys-Cys-Ala-NH_2

1

5 10
Arg-Asp-Cys-Cys-Thr-Hyp-Hyp-Arg-Lys-Cys-Lys-Asp-Arg-Arg-
15 20
Cys-Lys-Hyp-Met-Lys-Cys-Cys-Ala-NH_2

2

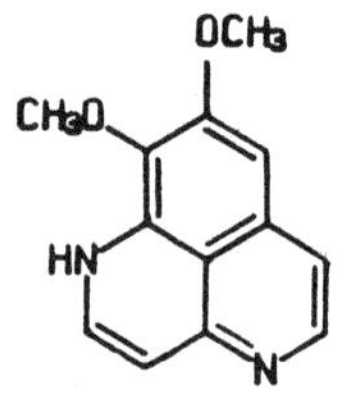

3

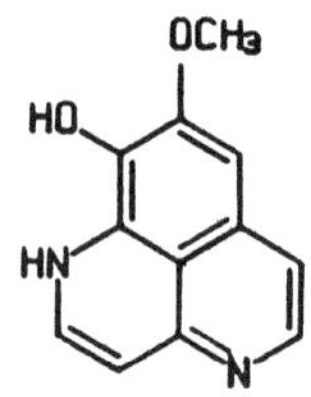

4

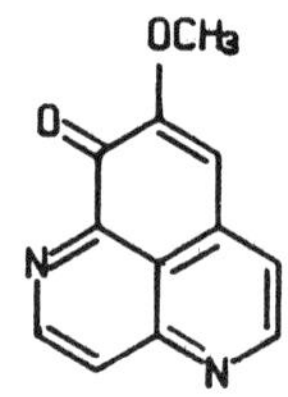

5

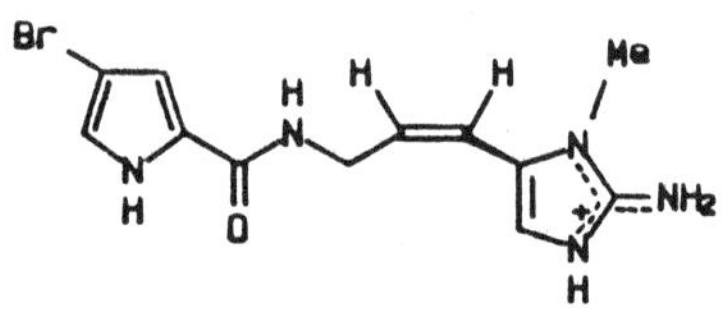

6

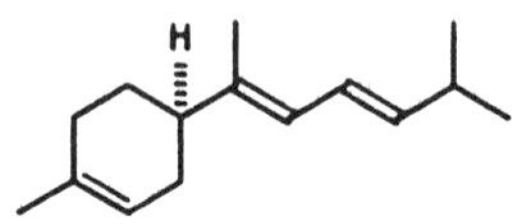

7

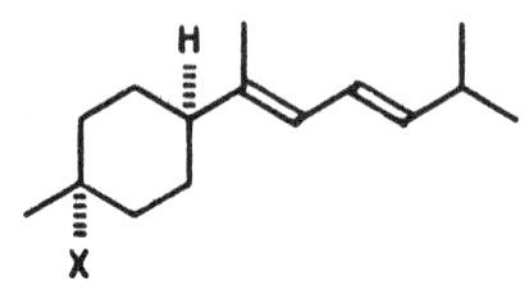

8 X=NHCHO
9 X=NCS

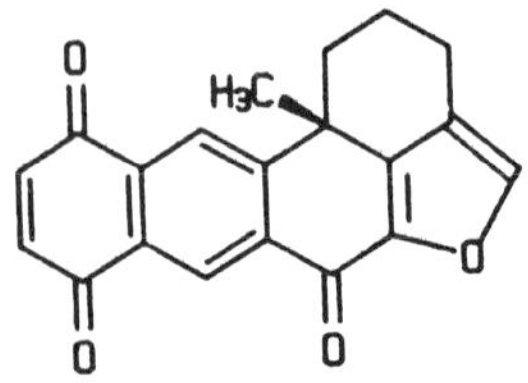

10

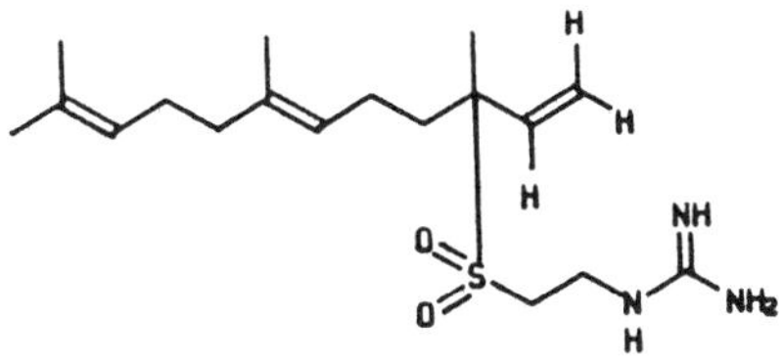

11

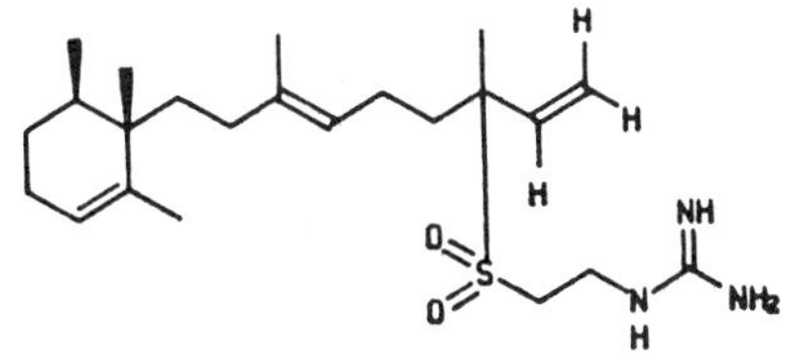

12

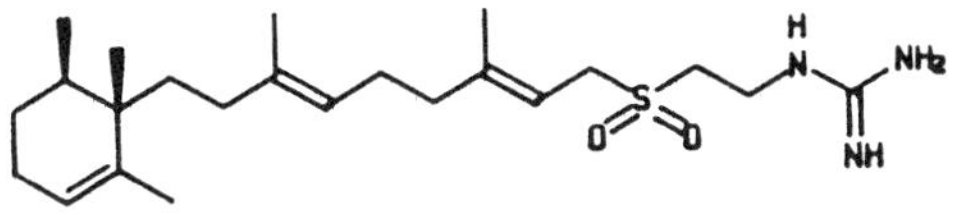

13

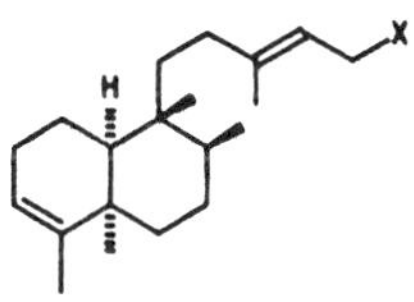

14

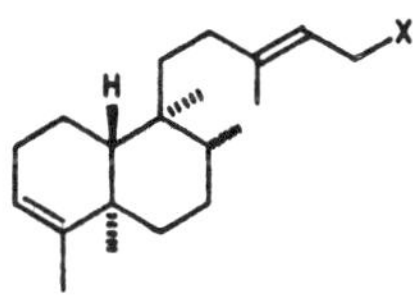

15

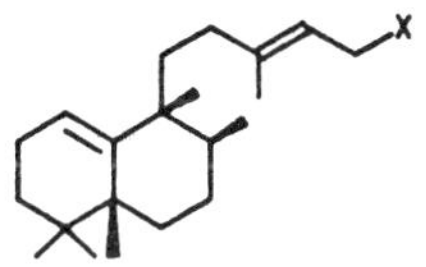

16

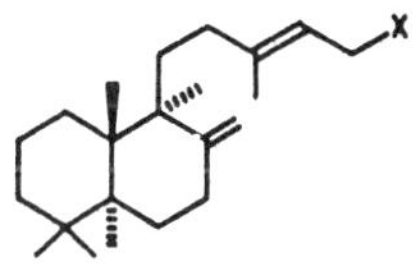

17

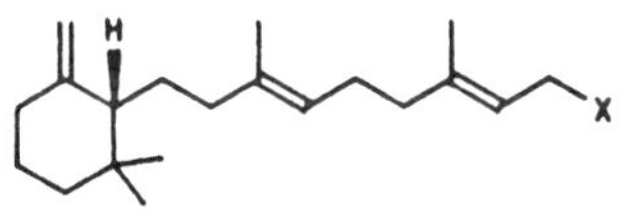

18

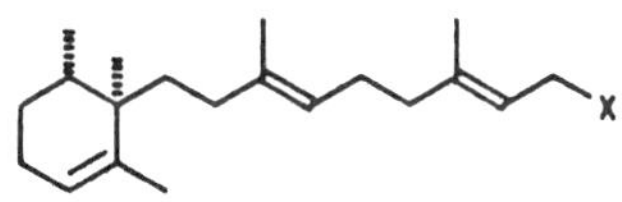

19

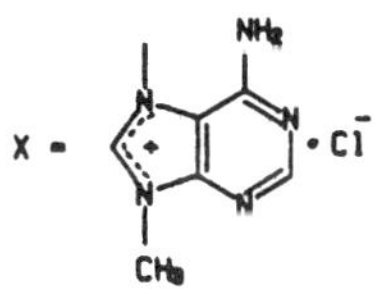

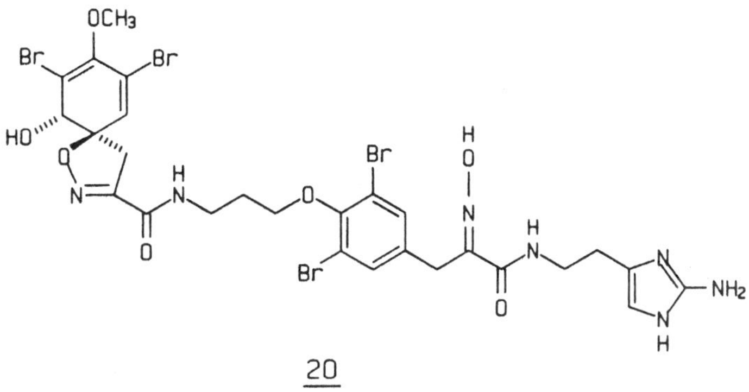

20

Eburnetoxin (mol wt, *ca.* 28,000)[9] and tessulatoxin (mol wt, 26,000),[10] powerful vasoactive proteins, have been isolated from the venoms of *C. eburneus* and *C. tessulatus*, respectively. These elicit the contractile response of the rabbit aorta, resulting from increased verapamil-sensitive calcium permeability across the smooth muscle membrane. The venom extract of *C. textile* caused a marked contraction in the guinea pig ileum and yielded a large amount of arachidonic acid as the active principle.[11,12]

Bioactive Metabolites from Marine Sponges. Marine sponges frequently produce large quantities of bioactive secondary metabolites that are thought to deter predators and to inhibit the growth of fouling organisms. In our bioassay system the 70% ethanol extracts of several sponge species exhibited marked activities, which we followed to isolate the active substances from their extracts.

The marine sponge *Aaptos aaptos* contained large amounts of new alkaloids--aaptamine (3) having α-adrenoceptor blocking activity,[13] and cytotoxic demethylaaptamine (4) and demethyloxyaaptamine (5). We prepared their derivatives and studied the contribution of functional groups in the aaptamine molecule to the α-adrenoceptor blocking activity.[14] The aromatic tricyclic ring system and the methoxy group of aaptamine may play an important role in the development of α-adrenoceptor blocking activity.

Keramadine (6), a bromopyrrole antagonist of the serotonergic receptor of the rabbit aorta,[15] was isolated from the marine sponge *Agelas nemoechinata*. Theonellin (7) and related compounds 8 and 9 were isolated from the sponge *Theonella* cf. *swinhoei*.[16]

Xestoquinone (10), a novel pentacyclic quinone isolated from the marine sponge *Xestospongia sapra*, inhibited cyclic AMP phosphodiesterase, elevating the intracellular cyclic AMP level, and thus causing a powerful cardiotonic effect.[17] The related known compound, halenaquinone, isolated from the same sponge, showed cardiotonic activity several times weaker than that of xestoquinone.

The antispasmodic agelasidines A, B, and C (11-13), isolated[18,19] from the marine sponge *Agelas nakamurai* inhibited the contraction of smooth muscles, the growth of microorganisms, and enzymic reactions of pig brain Na,K-ATPase. Furthermore, 9-methyladenine derivatives, agelasines A, B, C, D, E, and F (14-19) were obtained.[20,21] The agelasines and agelasidines were assayed for inhibition of Na,K-ATPase. The hydrophobic terpenoid part and the polar unit were important to the activity.

Purealin (20) and lipopurealins are Na,K-ATPase inhibitors obtained from the marine sponge *Psammaplysilla purea*.[22] Lipopurealins inhibited myosin Ca-ATPase and K,EDTA-ATPase from rabbit skeletal muscle as well as pig brain Na,K-ATPase. However, purealin activated myosin K,EDTA-ATPase and enhanced superprecipitation of myosin B. Purealin is the first example of an activator of myosin K,EDTA-ATPase. A study is under way to compare their effects on pharmacologically important enzymes with their effects on mammalian muscle preparations.

Bioactive Metabolites from Soft Corals and Tunicates. During a survey of *ca.* 50 species of Okinawan soft corals, a Ca-antagonistic diterpene, deoxysarcophine (21), was isolated from the soft coral *Sarcophyton* sp. and its structure established by X-ray analysis.[23] This is the first example of a terpenoid Ca-antagonist of marine or terrestrial origin.

Purification of several antimicrobial compounds from Okinawan tunicates is being carried out. Some of those tunicates also exhibit interesting pharmacological activity in mammalian muscle preparations.

UV-Absorbing Substances from Marine Organisms. A series of novel amino acids with strong UV absorption maxima in the range 310-360 nm has been isolated from marine plants and animals, the physiological roles of these substances, however, remain uncertain. In the course of our marine research we isolate numerous related compounds (22-

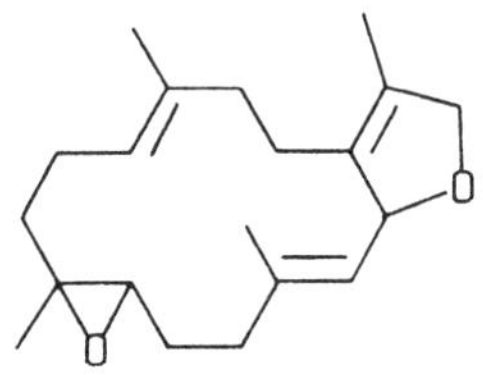

21

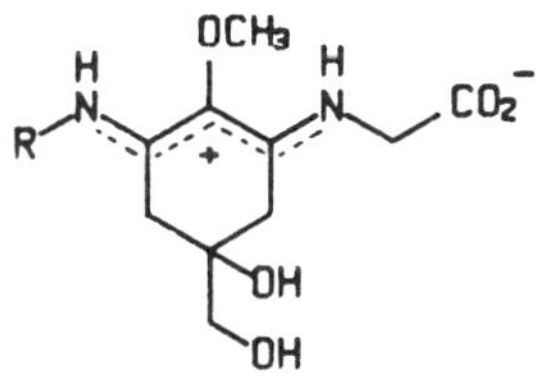

OCH3
H
N
R
CO2⁻
+
OH
OH

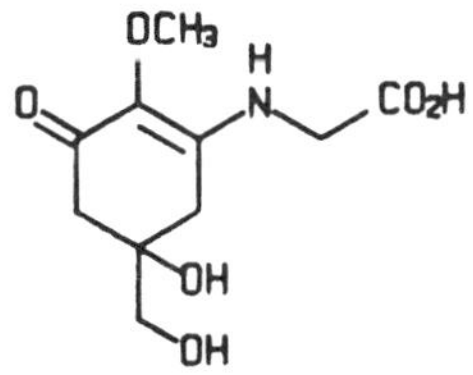

OCH3
H
N
O
CO2H
OH
OH

30

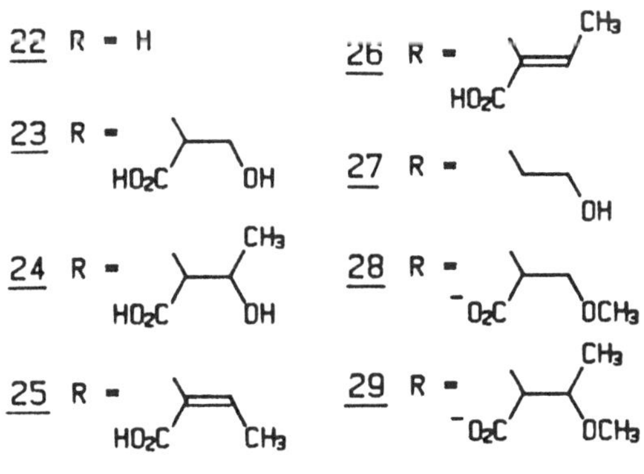

22 R = H
23 R =
HO2C
OH
24 R =
CH3
HO2C
OH
25 R =
HO2C
CH3
26 R =
CH3
HO2C
27 R =
OH
28 R =
⁻O2C
OCH3
29 R =
CH3
⁻O2C
OCH3

30) having characteristic UV absorption from the red algae *Halymenia florensia* and *Galaxaura fastigiata*, the ascidian *Halocynthia roretzi*,[24] the starfish *Asterina pectinifera*,[25] and the sea anemone *Radianthus* sp. We studied their distribution and composition in a variety of marine organisms and established that these substances are widespread among marine invertebrates and algae.[26] On the other hand, no significant pharmacological activity has been found among those UV-absorbing compounds subjected thus far to our bioassay system.

REFERENCES

1. Kobayashi, J.; Nakamura, H.; Hirata, Y.; Ohizumi, Y., *Toxicon*, 1982, *20*, 823.
2. Nakamura, H.; Kobayashi, J.; Ohizumi, Y.; Hirata, Y., *Experientia*, 1983, *39*, 590.
3. Sato, S.; Nakamura, H.; Ohizumi, Y.; Kobayashi, J.; Hirata, Y., *FEBS Lett.*, 1983, *155*, 277.
4. Nakamura, H.; Sato, S.; Kobayashi, J.; Ohizumi, Y.; Hirata, Y., in *Peptide Chemistry*, E. Munekata, Ed., Protein Research Foundation, Osaka, 1984, pp 197-202.
5. Kobayashi, J.; Nakamura, H.; Ohizumi, Y., *Br. J. Pharmac.*, 1981, *73*, 583.
6. Kobayashi, J.; Nakamura, H.; Hirata, Y.; Ohizumi, Y., *Biochem. Biophys. Res. Commun.*, 1982, *105*, 1389.
7. Kobayashi, J.; Nakamura, H. Ohizumi, Y., *Toxicon*, 1985, *23*, 783.
8. Kobayashi, J. Nakamura, H.; Ohizumi, Y., *Eur. J. Pharmac.*, 1983, *86*, 283.
9. Kobayashi, J., Nakamura, H.; Hirata, Y. Ohizumi, Y., *Life Sci.*, 1982, *31*, 1085.
10. Kobayashi, J.; Nakamura, H., Hirata, Y.; Ohizumi, Y., *Comp. Biochem. Physiol.*, 1983, *74*, 381.
11. Kobayashi, J.; Ohizumi, Y.; Nakamura, H.; Hirata, Y., *Toxicon*, 1981, *19*, 757.
12. Nakamura, H.; Kobayashi, J.; Ohizumi, Y.; Hirata, Y., *Experientia*, 1982, *38*, 897.
13. Nakamura, H.; Kobayashi, J. Ohizumi, Y.; Hirata, Y., *Tetrahedron Lett.*, 1982, *23*, 5555.
14. Ohizumi, Y.; Kajiwara, A.; Nakamura, H.; Kobayashi, J., *J. Pharm. Pharmacol.*, 1984, *36*, 785.
15. Nakamura, H.; Ohizumi, Y.; Kobayashi, J.; Hirata, Y., *Tetrahedron Lett.*, 1984, *25*, 2475.
16. Nakamura, J.; Kobayashi, J.; Ohizumi, Y.; Hirata, Y., *Tetrahedron Lett.*, 1984, *25*, 5401.
17. Nakamura, H.; Kobayashi, J.; Kobayashi, M.; Ohizumi, Y.; Hirata, Y., *Chem. Lett.*, 1985, 713.
18. Nakamura, H.; Wu, H.; Kobayashi, J.; Ohizumi, Y.; Hirata, Y.; Higashijima, T.; Miyazawa, T., *Tetrahedron Lett.*, 1983, *24*, 4105.
19. Nakamura, H.; Wu, H.; Kobayashi, J.; Kobayashi, M.; Ohizumi, Y.; Hirata, Y., *J. Org. Chem.*, 1985, *50*, 2494.
20. Nakamura, H.; Wu, H.; Ohizumi, Y.; Hirata, Y., *Tetrahedron Lett.*, 1984, *25*, 2989.
21. Wu, H.; Nakamura, H.; Kobayashi, J.; Ohizumi, Y.; Hirata, Y., *Tetrahedron Lett.*, 1984, *25*, 3719.
22. Nakamura, H.; Wu, H.; Kobayashi, J. Nakamura, Y.; Ohizumi, Y.; Hirata, Y., *Tetrahedron Lett.*, 1985, *26*, 4517.
23. Kobayashi, J.; Ohizumi, Y.; Nakamura, H.; Yamakado, T.; Matsuzaki, T.; Hirata, Y., *Experientia*, 1983, *39*, 67.
24. Kobayashi, J.; Nakamura, H.; Hirata, Y., *Tetrahedron Lett.*, 1981, *22*, 3001.
25. Nakamura, H.; Kobayashi, J.; Hirata, Y., *Chem. Lett.*, 1981, 1413.
26. Nakamura, H.; Kobayashi, J.; Hirata, Y., *J. Chromatogr.*, 1982, *250*, 113.

Koji Nakanishi
Suntory Institute for Bio-organic Research, Wakayamadai, Shimamoto-cho, Mishima-gun, Osaka 618, Japan *and*
Department of Chemistry, Columbia University, New York, New York 10027, U.S.A.

Marine Chemistry at Columbia University and the Suntory Institute for Bio-organic Research

SHARK-REPELLING PAVONININS[1] AND MOSESINS[2]

The pavoninins isolated from the shark-repelling South Pacific flat fish *Pardachirus pavoninus* are steroidal saponins containing glc-NAc as the sugar moiety (Figure 1). Recently, K. Tachibana at Sunbor identified four similar compounds, the "mosesins" from the Red Sea Moses sole *P. marmoratus*; they contain galactose as the sugar residue.[2] They all repel sharks, but their pharmacological activities may be even more interesting. Molecular models show the top of the steroid molecule to be hydrophobic whereas the bottom is very hydrophilic because of dangling sugar moieties. Such model steroids, as well as some mosesins, will be synthesized for field tests with sharks and for pharmacological assays. Recently, shark-repelling, 33-residue peptides also isolated from these flat fish have been synthesized. The size of these peptides makes them suitable for physicochemical studies of their tertiary structures and for syntheses of analogues.

CRUSTACEAN MOLTING INHIBITING HORMONE (MIH)[3]

The so-called X organ of crustacean eye stalks secretes a hormone that inhibits the biosynthesis of ecdysone by the Y organ. For the past six years, Y. Naya has been involved at Sunbor with the isolation and characterization of MIH. A compound isolated in minute quantities from the active fraction was assigned a structure, but unfortunately a synthetic sample lacked MIH activity. The great challenge of this problem, which has eluded all past isolation attempts, lies in the bioassay, that is, in securing Y organs that produce ecdysones. Studies in this area will continue.

SEA ANEMONE FISH SYMBIOSIS PROMOTER[4]

Y. Naya, M. Murata, and K. Kohshima have recently been able to characterize the substances responsible for the symbiosis between the sea anemone and the clown-fish. This is the first time such symonomes from sea water have been isolated and characterized.

TUNICHROME[5]

An even greater challenge than characterization of unidentified TB-1 congeners is the clarification of the biological roles of tunichromes and vanadium, and the determination

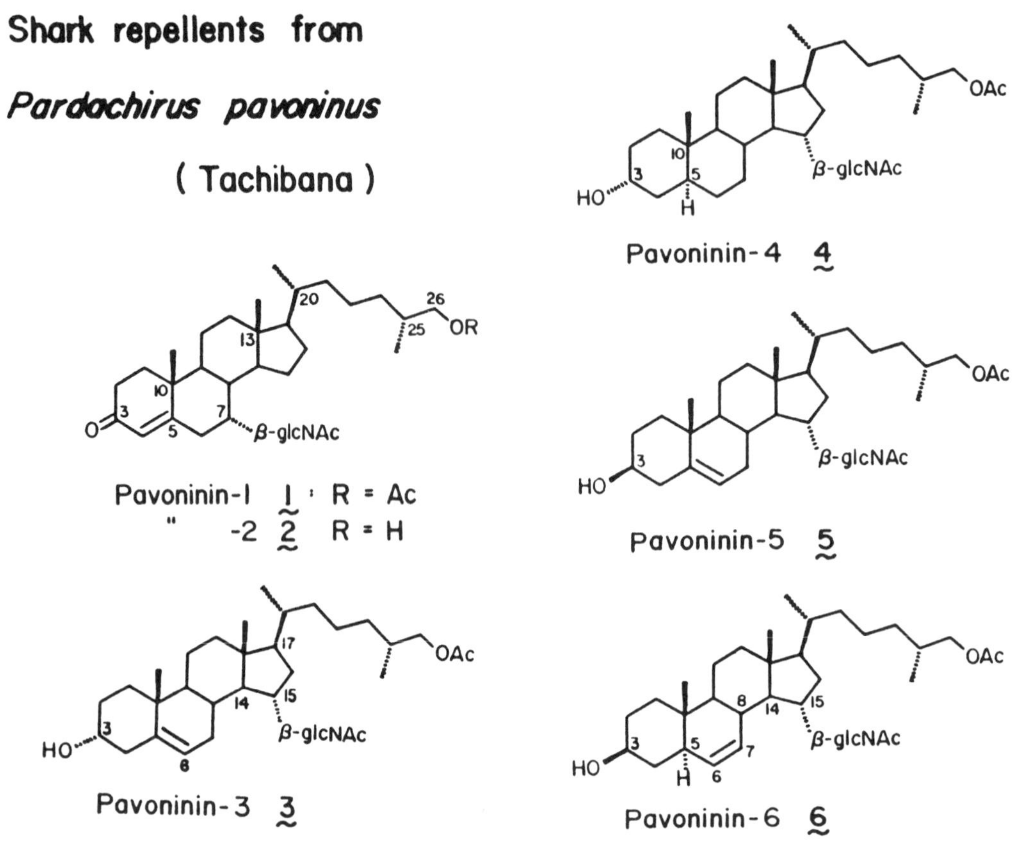

Figure 1

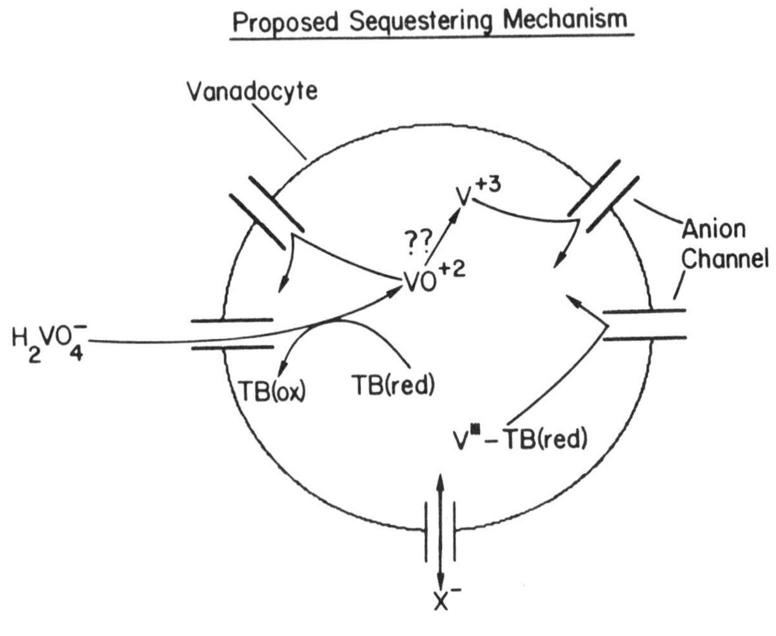

Figure 2

Toxins from *Ptychodiscus brevis*

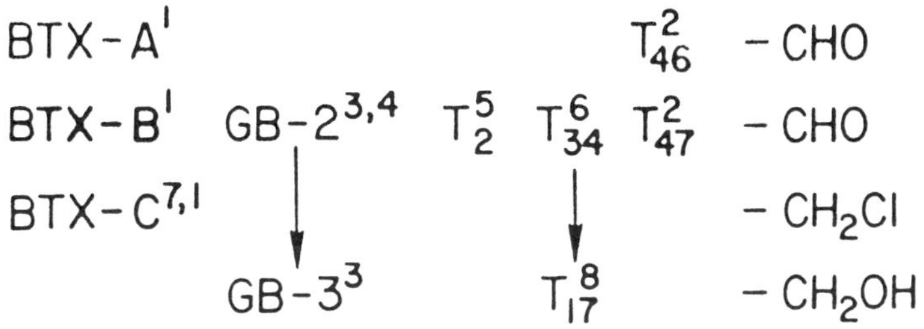

1. Lin, et al., *JACS,* 6773 (81)
2. Risk, et al., "*Toxic Din. Blooms,*" 351 (79)
3. Chou, Shimizu, *TL,* 5521 (82)
4. Shimizu, "*Marine Nat. Prod.,*" I, 1 (78)
5. Alam, et al., *J. Pharm. Sci.,* 865 (75)
6. Baden, et al., *Toxicon,* 455 (81)
7. Golik, et al., *TL,* 2535 (82)
8. Baden, Mende, *Toxicon,* 452 (82)

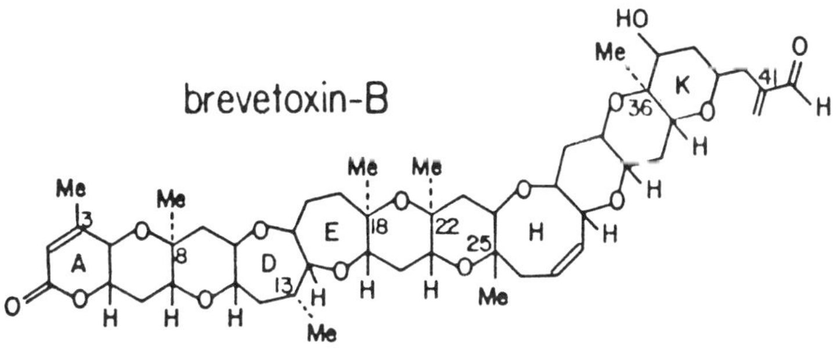

Figure 3

of the oxidation state of vanadium in the blood. The phase diagram of vanadium, which has oxidation states ranging from +5 to -1, is extremely complex; while it is generally believed to exist 90% as vanadium(III) and 10% as vanadium(IV), this has not been proven. Both vanadium(III) and vanadium(IV) precipitate above pH 3, but clearly vanadium is dissolved in blood at *ca.* neutral pH, probably because it is complexed with the tunichrome in some unknown way.

Once it is in the blood, vanadium is known to accumulate further, reaching concentrations of 1 molar in adults. We may hypothesize that vanadium, which exists in sea water as the pentavalent oxyanion $H_2VO_4^-$ (vanadate), enters the blood cells through an anion gate; once in the cell, it is immediately reduced to vanadium(IV) by the strongly reducing tunichromes. Neither vanadium(IV) nor vanadium(III) cations can be released through the anion channel and hence they accumulate (Figure 2).

The isolation of tunichrome was not easy and the tunichrome project demonstrates the fact that structure determination is only a first step toward understanding the structural basis of life mechanisms. Mode-of-action studies will be far more difficult and challenging, but they should be possible as new techniques become available to natural product chemists.

BREVETOXINS[6]

In 1981 we were able to purify the brevetoxins (BTX), the red-tide toxins responsible for massive fish kills, and to determine the structure of one of them, BTX-B.[6,7] Here again, the toxins were known since 1968 but were not purified despite considerable interest in them as neurotoxins which open the sodium channel.[8] Several more BTXs were characterized after BTX-B (Figure 3). Our current efforts deal with several aspects of the brevetoxins: (1) the unique, unprecedented BTX skeleton, an interesting target for biosynthetic studies, which are being carried out with ^{13}C-labeled precursors; (2) the structure of BTX-A, which has a different skeleton and thus far has not been obtained in crystalline form suitable for X-ray studies; (3) attachment of the diazoacetoxy group as a photoaffinity label to appropriate hydroxyl groups in order to bind the toxins to the sodium channel; (4) increased production by the BTX-producing dinoflagellate *Ptychodiscus brevis* so that BTX can be made available in milligram quantities.

REFERENCES

1. Tachibana, K.; Sakaitani, M.; Nakanishi, K., *Sciences*, 1984, *226*, 703; *Tetrahedron*, 1985, *41*, 1027; Tachibana, K., in "Toxins, Drugs, and Pollutants in Marine Animals", Bolis, L. *et al.*, Eds., Springer Verlag, Berlin and Heidelberg, 1984, pp 2-12.
2. Thompson, S.A.; Tachibana, K.; Nakanishi, K.; Kubota, I., *Science (Washington, D.C.)*, 1986, *233*, 341; Tachibana, K.; *et al.*, to be published.
3. Naya, Y.; *et al.*, unpublished.
4. Murata, M.; Miyagawa-Kohshima, K.; Nakanishi, K.; Naya, Y., *Science (Washington, D.C.)*, 1986, *234*, 585; Murata, M.; *et al.*, to be published.
5. Bruening, R.C.; Oltz, E.M.; Furukawa, J.; Nakanishi, K.; Kustin, K., *J. Am. Chem. Soc.*, 1985, *107*, 5298; *J. Nat. Prod.*, 1986, *49*, 193.
6. Lin, Y.Y.; Risk, M.; Ray, S.M.; Van Engen, D.; Golik, J.; James, J.C.; Nakanishi, K., *J. Am. Chem. Soc.*, 1981, *103*, 6773.
7. Nakanishi, K., *Toxicon*, 1985, *23*, 473.
8. "Toxic Dinoflagellate Blooms", D.L. Taylor and H.H. Seliger, Eds., New York, NY, Elsevier/North Holland, 1979.

Luigi Minale
Dipartimento di Chimica delle Sostanze Naturali, Università, Via L. Rodinò 22, 80138 Napoli, Italy

Marine Natural Products Research at Laboratories in Naples, Italy

I shall review here the research activity during the past fifteen years in marine natural products chemistry at the University of Naples and at the National Research Council (C.N.R.) Laboratories in Naples, with special emphasis on continuing research programs.

The tradition of marine research in Naples began in 1872 when Anton Dohrn founded the Zoological Station, which has been a base for many prestigious researchers in marine biology. Today, the Station still plays an important role in marine science, and its presence in the scientific culture of Naples has stimulated interest in the study of natural compounds from marine organisms. A C.N.R. Laboratory for the Chemistry of Molecules of Biological Interest was established in 1969 at Arco Felice near Naples; its first director (1969-1973), Professor R.A. Nicolaus, strongly encouraged marine research. Professor Nicolaus's most important contributions concerned the chemistry of melanins, pigments present in a variety of biological systems ranging from the integuments and body fluids of various invertebrates to mammalian hair, skin, and eyes. Interestingly, most of the knowledge about the structure of these natural melanins is derived from Nicolaus's studies of the black pigment, sepiomelanin, isolated from the ink sac of the cuttlefish *Sepia officinalis*. Thus, the decision made by a group of us at Naples to direct our attention toward the chemistry of marine natural products was also aimed at continuing a tradition.

When the new C.N.R. opened in 1969, Professor E. Fattorusso and I, with a group of younger colleagues (G. Cimino, S. De Stefano, and G. Sodano, joined later by R. Riccio and S. De Rosa) began to study extracts from *Verongia aerophoba*, a common yellow sponge in the bay of Naples, with a view to isolating and identifying its pigments. The unexpected discovery in remarkable yields of aerothionin and the aeroplysinins, brominated antibiotics biogenetically related to 3,5-dibromotyrosine, prompted a systematic research for new products from Mediterranean sponges.

Between 1970 and 1977 more than fifty species of the class Demospongiae were examined at Arco Felice for their secondary metabolites. About one hundred new molecules were discovered, most of them terpenes with unique structures. Among the brominated metabolites, aeroplysinin-1 (1)[1] has received the most attention because of its antitumor activity in KB cells and in L1210 leukemia assays.

Among sesquiterpenoids I would like to mention avarol (2),[2] a sesquiterpenoid hydroquinone with a rearranged drimane skeleton and significant antitumor activity *in vivo*.

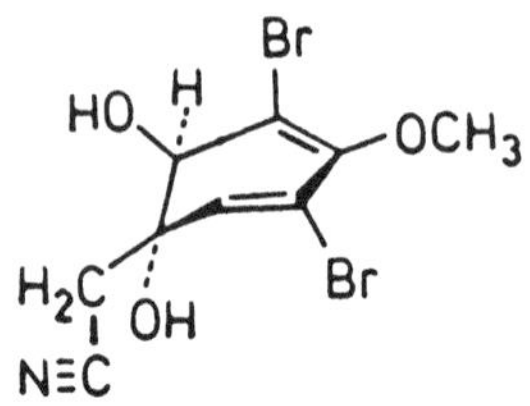

1

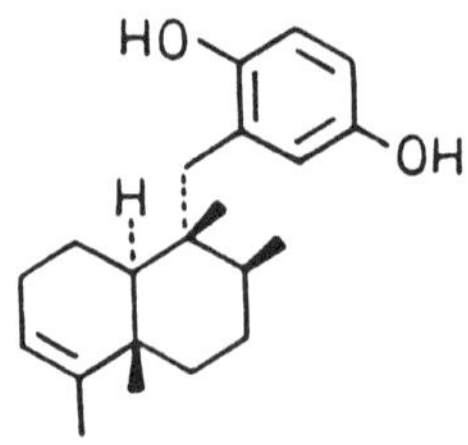

2

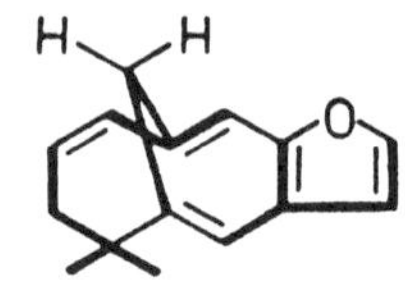

3

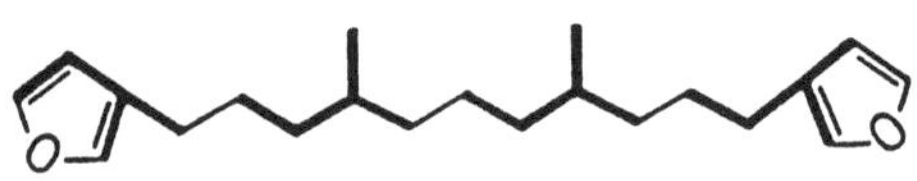

4

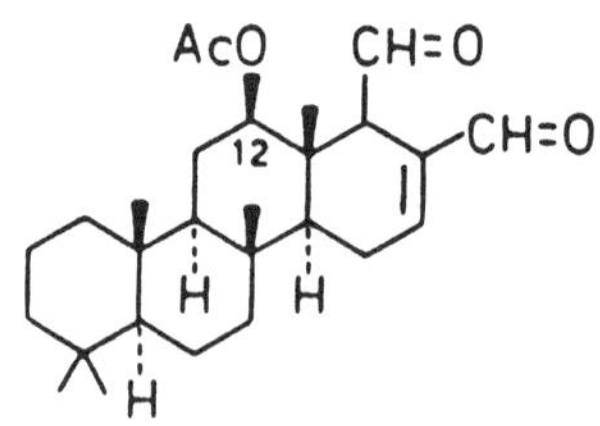

5

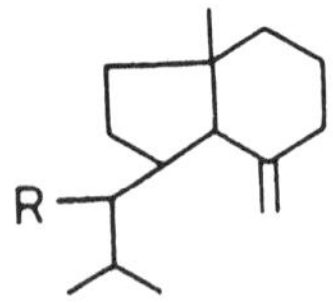

6 R=N⁺≡C⁻

7 R=N=C=S

8 R=NHCH=O

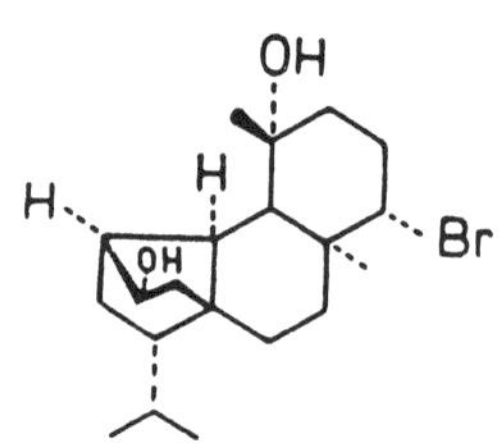

9

The interesting pharmaceutical and biological activities of avarol are being investigated by German and Yugoslav workers (W.E.G. Müller, D. Sladic, and their colleagues), who reported both the inhibition of mitosis and alteration of DNA by avarol at the IUPAC Fifth Symposium on Marine Natural Products (Paris, September 1985).

Of the vast array of sesquiterpene furans isolated from sponges at Arco Felice, the very unstable spiniferin-1 (3) is, at present, the only sesquiterpene known to have the 1,6-methano-[10]-annulene carbon skeleton,[3] recently confirmed by total synthesis.[4] The linear C_{21} difurans (4) are intriguing compounds from a biogenetic point of view. They probably arise from sesterterpenes formed by successive head-to-tail additions of five isoprene units and are relatively abundant in sponges. A clue to the biosynthetic route was provided by the discovery in certain species of *Ircinia* of both C_{21} and C_{25} metabolites. Some of the linear C_{21} and C_{25} furanoterpenes have antimicrobial activity.

The scalarins, tetracyclic sesterterpenes that are relatively common in Dictyoceratid sponges,[5] are particularly interesting because some of them are cytotoxic.[6] M. Endo of the Suntory Institute for Biomedical Research recently drew attention to this group of compounds by reporting potent hypotensive activity of 12-*epi*-scalaradial (5).[7]

Finally, the Naples laboratory has contributed to knowledge of the "non-conventional" sterols of sponges. Aplysterol and didehydroaplysterol, discovered at Arco Felice, were the first examples of C-26-alkylation in steroid biosynthesis,[8] and the 19-nor- and A-nor-sterols were studied later.[9] Fattorusso and colleagues discovered calysterol with a unique cyclopropene ring in the side chain,[10] and more recently, Sica *et al.* isolated petrosterol, another cyclopropane-containing sterol.[11]

These examples indicated that sponges may be sources of new types of sterols and prompted a systematic search. An extraordinary number of new sterols with remarkable side chain alkylation patterns were discovered, especially by Professor Djerassi. Results obtained in the period 1970-1977 are reviewed in several monographs (*e.g.*, Refs. 12 and 13).

In 1972 Professor Fattorusso returned to the Institute of Organic Chemistry of the University of Naples, where Professor Prota began to study the pigmentation chemistry of marine invertebrates. Later in 1977 I also moved to the University's Institute for Bioorganic Chemistry (now the Department of Chemistry of Natural Products). Thus, three University groups joined the Arco Felice group, now under the leadership of Drs. Cimino and Sodano, in the fascinating adventure of marine natural products. One more group was established at Catania under the leadership of Professor Piattelli.

The establishment in Italy in 1980 of a national research project, Progretto Finalizzato, "Chimica Fine e Secondaria", sponsored by the C.N.R., gave all five groups the opportunity to collaborate and use common facilities. For example, "Progetto Finalizzato" arranged for Farmitalia-Carlo Erba, a national pharmaceutical industry, to subject compounds isolated from marine organisms to a series of pharmacological tests--central nervous system, angiotension-converting enzyme, antiulcer, immunomodulatory, antiallergic, antimicrobial, antiviral, and *in vivo* antitumoral assays. Of more than one hundred marine compounds tested by Farmitalia-Carlo Erba, a relatively large number have antimicrobial activity, several are cytotoxic, some are hypotensive agents, and one is antiviral.

The contributions of the Neapolitan groups and their current programs are outlined below.

Professor E. Fattorusso's group (D. Sica, C. Santacroce, L. Mayol, S. Magno, L. De Napoli, and F. Cafieri) of the Dipartimento di Chimica delle Sostanze Naturali, Università, Napoli, have continued the search for sponge metabolites. They have isolated a large number of novel terpenoids, some of them possessing rare isocyanide, isothiocyanate, and formamide groups, as exemplified by axisonitrile-1 (6), axisothiocyanate-1 (7), and axamide-1 (8), the first compounds of this series isolated.[14] Naturally occurring isonitriles are now firmly established as sponge metabolites, and their biological functions have been clarified to some extent.

In extensive collaborative efforts, Professors Piattelli at Catania and Fattorusso at Naples have carried out a systematic investigation of secondary metabolites of algae, and have discovered a great number of novel terpenoids, mostly diterpenoids. They have also been involved in the search for novel amino acids from algae; the work is described in the excellent monograph "Aminoacids from Marine Algae".[15]

In recent years the group has continued to focus on the structural organic chemistry of marine metabolites from sponges, algae, and hydroids. The problems involved are best illustrated by the recently determined structures 9 and 10. Coronopifoliol (9), from the alga *Sphaerococcus coronopifolius*, contains a unique carbocyclic ring system, which has been suggested to be biogenetically related to bromosphaerol, the major diterpene of the same alga.[16] Gracilin B (10), an interesting metabolite of the bis-nor-diterpene group, rare among marine products, was isolated from the sponge *Spongionella gracilis*.[17]

Professor G. Prota's group at the Dipartimento di Chimica Organica e Biologica, Università, Napoli, has continued the tradition of the Neapolitan school and has focused mainly on pigments. Hallachrome, a red pigment from the sea worm *Halla parthenopeia*, was assigned the unique 1,2-anthraquinone structure in 1972;[18] that structure elucidation began at the Zoological Station of Naples in 1930 when Mazza and Stolfi believed the pigment to be an indole-5,6-quinone derivative.

Prota and his associates have made important contributions to the chemistry of zoanthoxanthins, a novel group of yellow nitrogenous pigments distributed among anthozoans of the order Zoanthidea. Their structures include the unique diaminotetrazacyclopentazulene chromophore, either linear or angular (*i.e.* the zoanthoxanthin (11) and pseudozoanthoxanthin (12) series).[19]

Even more interesting is the study of adenochrome, an iron-sequestering pigment first reported in 1908, that confers a characteristic purple color on the branchial hearts of *Octopus vulgaris*. Early investigations did not proceed well and the subject remained dormant until 1943 when the pigment was discovered independently by Fox and Updeyrapp, who named it adenochrome. In 1974 Nardi and Steinberg re-isolated adenochrome from *O. vulgaris* and demonstrated definitively that the pigment is bound to Fe(III). In 1976 Prota developed an improved isolation procedure involving immediate and complete conversion of the material to the colorless deferriadenochrome. Extensive degradative studies have shown that the product is a complex mixture of related peptides derived from glycine and three novel amino acids; the adenochromines (13-15) arise biogenetically by addition of a hitherto unknown 5-histidinethiol to dopaquinone which accounts for the chelate formation with Fe(III).[19,20] Numerous attempts to define the sequence of the peptide chain have been hampered by unfavorable solubility properties of adenochrome(s) as well as by the structural complexity of adenochromines. Degradative experiments coupled with model biochemical synthesis, however, allowed formulation of a partial structure consisting of a hexapeptide formed by two adenochromylglycylglycine units.[21] Work is in progress to assess the potential usefulness of adenochrome(s) as new natural chelating agent(s) in the treatment of certain diseases such as Thalassemia mediterranea. Recently, significant amounts of 5-histidinethiol, a component of adenochrome(s), have been found as free amino acids in the eggs of sea urchins and other invertebrates.[22] This is of interest in relation to the known pharmacological activity of sulfydryl compounds.

The Arco Felice Group, Cimino and Sodano and their associates (De Stefano, De Rosa, Spinella) at the Istituto per la Chimica di Molecole d'Interesse Biologico del C.N.R. have concentrated on three main topics: (a) metabolites from sponges, (b) marine zoochromes,

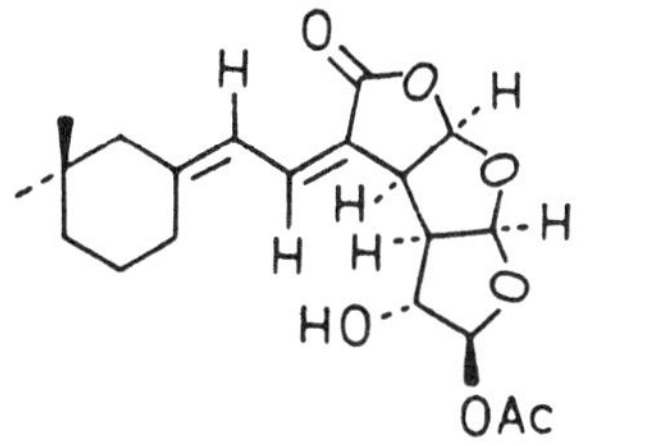

10

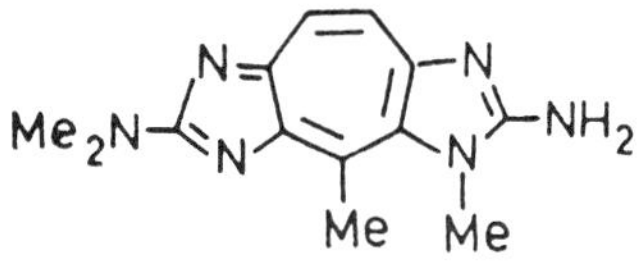

11

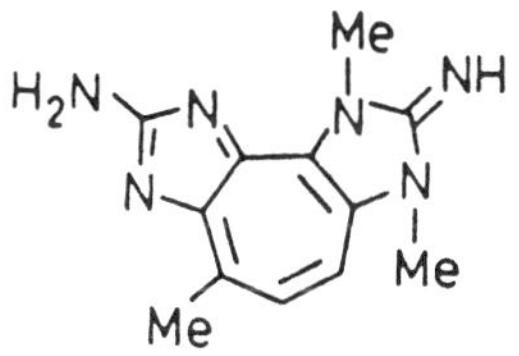

12

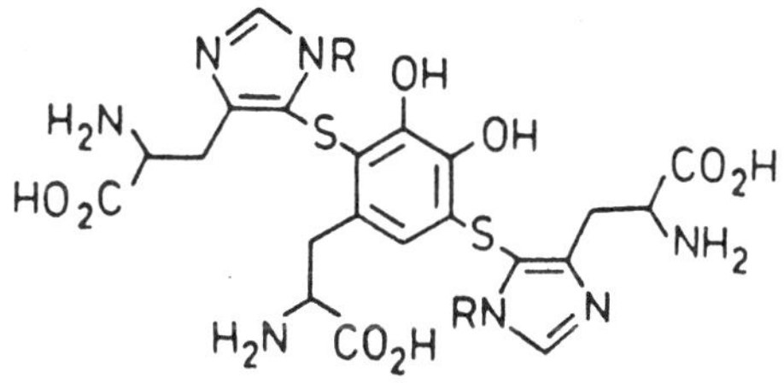

13

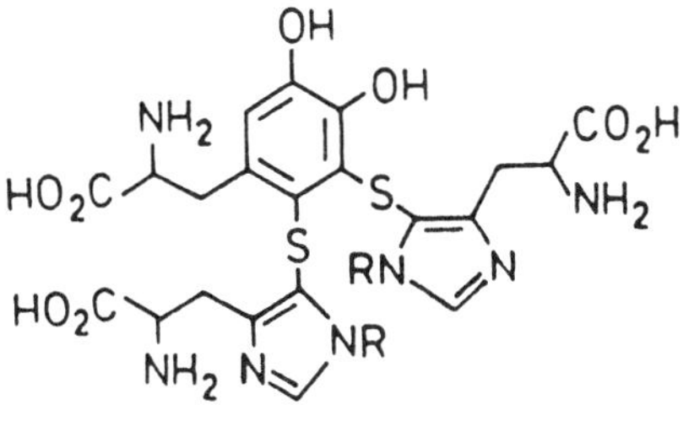

14

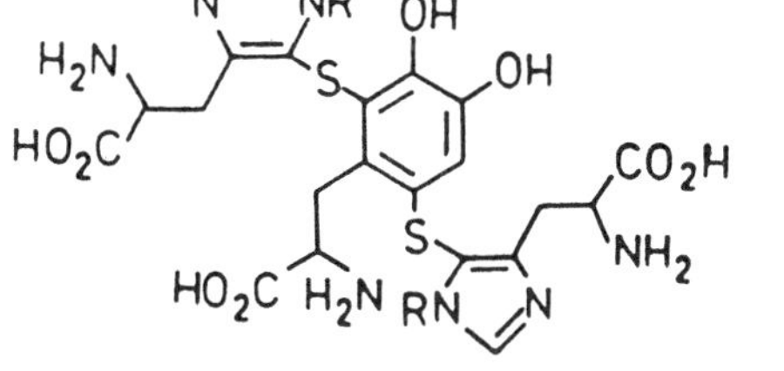

15

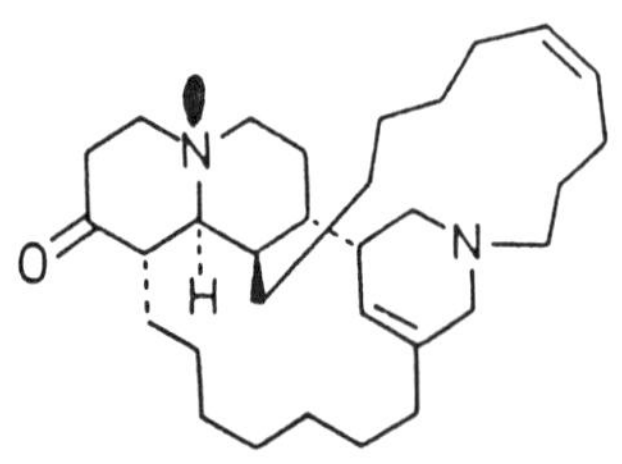

16

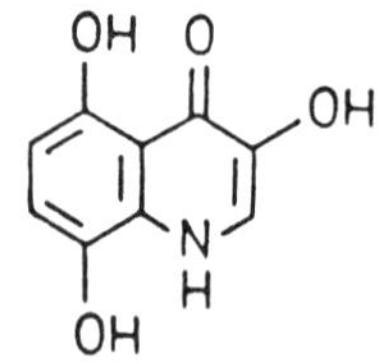

17

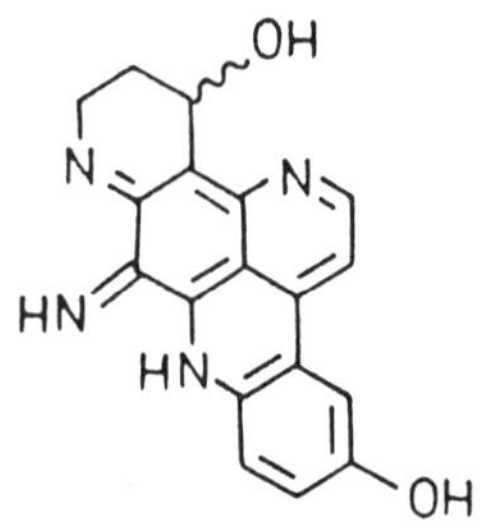

18

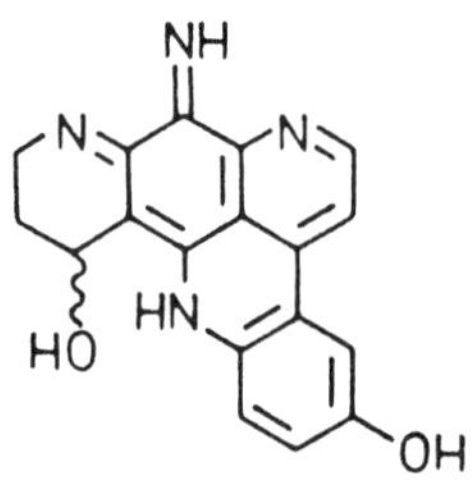

19

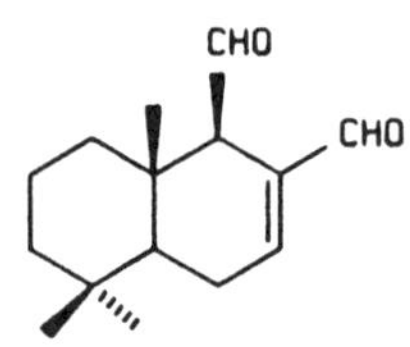

20

and (c) the defensive behavior of Mediterranean opistobranchs. The most recent success in the first category concerned the structural elucidation of the sarains, homologous alkaloids from the sponge *Reniera sarai*. Interest in these compounds began in 1970, but only recently was an isolation procedure developed to avoid problems due to the formation of complexes with the salts present in the chromatographic materials. Extensive and detailed spectroscopic analysis, including the use of 2-D NMR, allowed Cimino and colleagues[23] to propose the structure 16 for sarain-1, with quinolizidine and tetrahydropyridine rings connected by two long alkyl chains. Sarains are moderately toxic and showed antiarrhythmic effects. The capacity to form stable complexes with salts gives the sarains properties comparable to those of the crown ethers. It is worth noting that the structures of other quinolizidine alkaloids from sponges have recently been described. A number of related metabolites from *Reniera sarai* are now being investigated at Arco Felice.

Recent advances in spectroscopic methods induced Cimino, Sodano and colleagues to undertake structural studies of complex molecules that resisted previous chemical investigations, among them the unstable zoochromes from the sponge *Verongia aerophoba* and from the sea anemone *Calliactis parasitica* (order Actiniaria). Uranidine, the yellow pigment of *V. aerophoba*, described for the first time a century ago, has the relatively simple structure 3,5,8-trihydroxy-4-quinolone (17), and is easily oxidized to the corresponding 5,8-quinone. The rapid polymerization of this quinone accounts for the blackening of the sponge on exposure to air.[24] Calliactine, the pigment of *Calliactis parasitica*, was reported in 1940 by E. Lederer and has a complex structure of a new skeletal type. Accurate spectroscopic analyses allowed Cimino and colleagues[23] to propose two alternative structures 18 and 19.

An intriguing and important area of marine natural products research is that which explains biological phenomena. The nudibranchs, which are characterized by the evolutionary loss of an external shell, have developed a series of defensive strategies, including the use of chemicals to deter predators. In a systematic search for defensive compounds of Mediterranean nudibranchs, Cimino and Sodano isolated a number of toxic antifeedant compounds and clarified many aspects of this problem. Some of the toxic compounds (*e.g.*, isocyanosesquiterpenes and furan sesquiterpenes) are of dietary origin, while antifeedant drimane sesquiterpenoids such as polygodial (20) are synthesized *de novo* by the animals. In their study of polygodial,[25] Cimino and Sodano provided the first evidence that a nudibranch, *Dendrodoris limbata*, can elaborate its own chemical defense. They also established that polygodial is stored in the mantle of the animal, while the digestive gland contains a series of sesquiterpenoid metabolites.[23,26] A convincing explanation for the bioactivity of polygodial has also been offered, relating its effect on the sense of taste by its ability to form adducts with -NH groups, rather than with -SH groups.[27] Extensive investigation of a group of similar dialdehydes has shown that the biological activities depend on the distance between the two aldehyde groups and on the size of the molecule.[28]

Since 1979 the Minale group (R. Riccio, C. Pizza and F. Zollo) at the Dipartimento di Chimica delle Sostanze Naturali, University of Naples, have been involved mainly with systematic research on the oligoglycosides found in starfishes (phylum Echinodermata). Sea cucumbers and starfish have been known to excrete saponin-like compounds, probably as part of a defense mechanism. Because the techniques for handling water-soluble saponins are so different from those generally employed in marine natural products chemistry, few groups have been involved in this type of research despite the many pharmacological properties ascribed to starfish and sea cucumber extracts. Our investigation of thirty Mediterranean and Pacific starfish species led to the isolation and structure elucidation of about fifty steroidal glycosides, which can be conveniently divided into three classes--sulfated steroidal glycosides; steroidal cyclic glycosides; and glycosides of

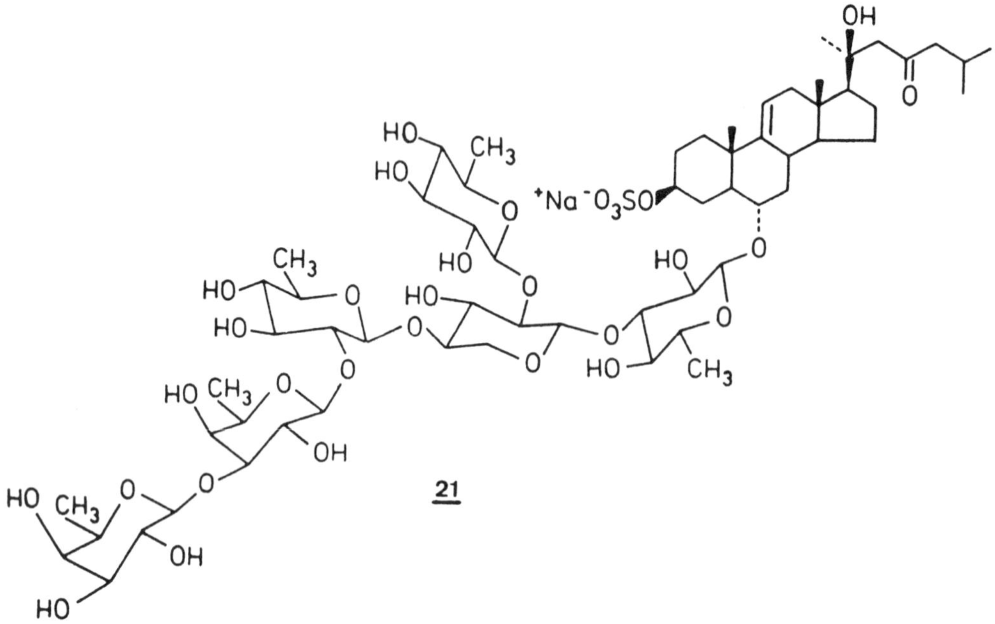

21

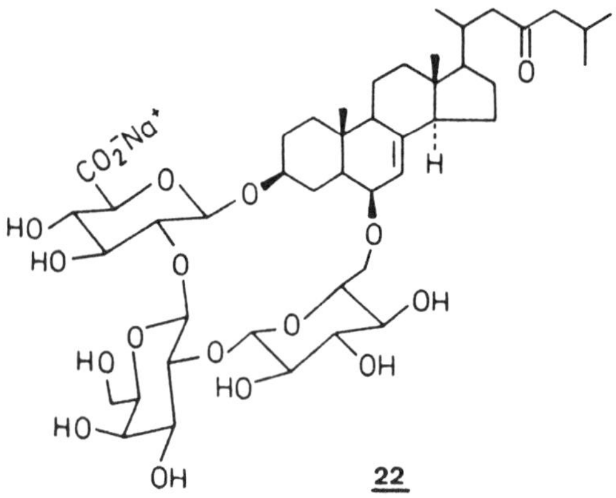

22

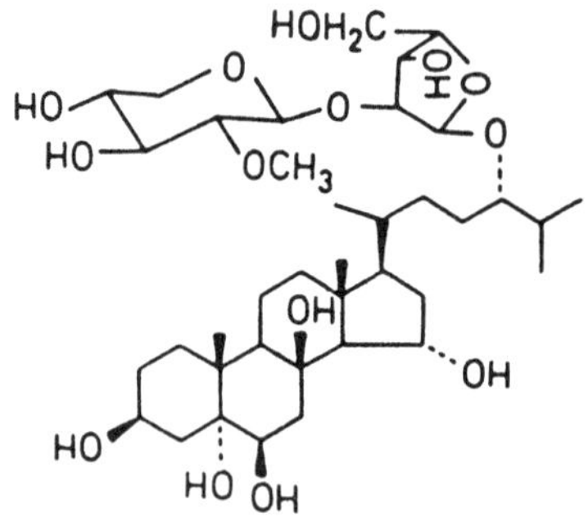

23

polyhydroxysteroids, consisting of a polyhydroxylated steroid with one or two sugar units.

The first group of glycosides, for which the term "asterosaponins" was originally coined, is present in all species examined except *Echinaster*, and many of the physiological and pharmacological activities reported for starfish extracts or purified fractions can be attributed to these compounds. All asterosaponins contain a $3\beta,6\alpha$-dihydroxy-Δ^{22}-steroidal moiety, an oligosaccharide attached at C-6, and a sulfate group at C-3. In the saccharide portion (five or six monosaccharide units) the interglycosidic linkages are also invariant, and the position of the branched unit is always located on the second monosaccharide unit starting from the aglycones. All sugars are in their pyranose form with the β-anomeric configuration. Marthasteroside A_2 (21)[29] has the general structure of such toxic saponins.

The toxic cyclic glycosides discovered in starfishes of the genus *Echinaster* do not have a sulfate group. They have unusual features such as a chain of three sugar units cyclized between C-3 and C-6 of the steroidal nucleus (*cf.* sepositoside A, 22, the major glycoside from *E. sepositus*).[30]

The structures of the third group of saponins, which usually occur in minute amounts, may be illustrated by the cytotoxic nodososide (23),[31] the first representative of such compounds. A recent survey of these results has been presented at the Naito International Symposium on Natural Products, Tokyo, November 1984.[32]

Our current research concerns metabolites from echinoderms (starfish, ophiuroid, and crinoid) and other invertebrates, with the main emphasis on water-soluble compounds. As Y. Shimizu pointed out,[33] water-soluble fractions from marine organisms have been grossly neglected, even though they contain such biologically active compounds as antineoplastic, cardiotonic, hypotensive and antimicrobial agents, as well as site-specific toxins, pheromones, hormones, and other allelochemicals. The tedious and time-consuming purification process is a major problem in handling water-soluble compounds, but recent advances in isolation techniques have enabled us to isolate some bioactive water-soluble compounds.

CONCLUSION

Marine natural product research in Naples has had two aims: (1) to contribute to the general knowledge of the chemistry and biology of marine organisms, and (2) to identify new pharmacological agents.

The first objective has been successfully achieved with an added contribution--the education and training of graduate students, postdoctoral fellows, and senior scientists. The competency developed over the years and the instrumental facilities currently available make Naples a well-established center in the field of the chemistry and biology of life processes.

Progress toward the second objective has been limited, partly because of the difficulties encountered in establishing fruitful collaborations with research teams dedicated to marine pharmacology. Research in marine chemistry will certainly continue in Naples, and better results in the search for new drugs of marine origin could be achieved through international, interdisciplinary collaborations. The research groups in Naples are eager to support such collaborations.

REFERENCES

1. Fattorusso, E.; Minale, L.; Sodano G., *J. Chem. Soc., Perkin Trans. I*, 1972, 16.

2. De Rosa, S.; Minale, L.; Riccio, R.; Sodano, G., *J. Chem. Soc., Perkin Trans. I*, 1976, 1408.
3. Cimino, G.; De Stefano, S.; Minale, L.; Trivellone, E., *Experientia*, 1978, *34*, 1425.
4. Marshall, J.A.; Conrow, R.E., *J. Am. Chem. Soc.*, 1983, *105*, 5679.
5. Fattorusso, E.; Magno, S.; Santacroce, C.; Sica, D., *Tetrahedron*, 1972, *28*, 6021; Cimino, G.; De Stefano, S.; Minale, L.; Trivellone, E., *J. Chem. Soc., Perkin Trans. I*, 1977, 1587.
6. Yasuda, F.; Teda, H., *Experientia*, 1981, *37*, 110.
7. Endo, M., lecture presented at the IUPAC Vth Symposium on Marine Natural Products, Paris, September 2-6, 1985.
8. De Luca, P.; De Rosa, M.; Minale, L.; Sodano, G., *J. Chem. Soc., Perkin Trans. I*, 1972, 2132.
9. Minale, L.; Sodano, G., *J. Chem. Soc., Perkin Trans. I*, 1974, 1888; *ibid.* 1974, 2380.
10. Fattorusso, E.; Magno, S.; Mayol, L.; Santacroce, C.; Sica, D., *Tetrahedron*, 1975, *31*, 1715.
11. Mattia, C.A.; Mazzarella, L.; Puliti, R.; Sica, D.; Zollo, F., *Tetrahedron Lett.*, 1978, 3953.
12. Minale, L.; Sodano, G.; De Stefano, S.; Sodano, G., *Fortschr. Chem. Org. Naturst.*, 1976, *33*, 1.
13. Minale, L., in *Marine Natural Products Chemical and Biological Perspectives*, P.J. Scheuer Ed., Academic Press, New York, 1978, Vol. I, p 175.
14. Cafieri, F.; Fattorusso, E.; Magno, S.; Santacroce, C.; Sica, D., *Tetrahedron*, 1973, *29*, 4259.
15. Fattorusso, E.; Piattelli, M., in *Marine Natural Products Chemical and Biological Perspectives*, J.P. Scheuer Ed., Academic Press, New York, 1980, Vol. III, p 95.
16. Cafieri, F.; Fattorusso, E.; Mayol, L.; Santacroce, C., *J. Org. Chem.*, 1985, *50*, 3982.
17. Mayol, L.; Piccialli, V.; Sica, D., *Tetrahedron Lett.*, 1985, *26*, 1253.
18. Prota, G.; D'Agostino, M.D.; Misuraca, G., *J. Chem. Soc., Perkin Trans. I*, 1972, 1614.
19. Prota, G., in *Marine Natural Products Chemical and Biological Perspectives*, P.J. Scheuer Ed., Academic Press, New York, 1980, Vol. III, p 141.
20. Prota, G.; Ito, S.; Nardi, G., in *Marine Natural Products*, J. Faulkner and W.H. Fenical Eds., Plenum Press, New York, 1977, p 45; Ito, S.; Nardi, G.; Palumbo, G.; Prota, G., *J. Chem. Soc., Perkin Trans. I*, 1979, 2617.
21. Prota, G., personal communication.
22. Palumbo, A.; Misuraca, G.; D'Ischia, M.; Donaudy, F.; Prota, G., *Comp. Biochem. Physiol.*, 1984, *78B*, 81.
23. Cimino, G.; De Rosa, S.; De Stefano, S.; Sodano, G., *Abstracts IUPAC Fifth International Symposium on Marine Natural Products*, Paris, September 2-6, 1985.
24. Cimino, G.; De Rosa, S.; De Stefano, S.; Spinella, A.; Sodano, G., *Tetrahedron Lett.* 1984, *25*, 2925.
25. Cimino, G.; De Rosa, S.; De Stefano, S.; Sodano, G.; Villani, G., *Science (Washington, D.C.)*, 1983, *219*, 1237.
26. Cimino, G.; De Rosa, S.; De Stefano, S.; Morrone, R.; Sodano, G., *Tetrahedron Lett.*, 1985, *26*, 1093.
27. D'Ischia, M.; Prota, G.; Sodano, G., *Tetrahedron Lett.*, 1982, *23*, 3295.
28. Cimino, G.; Spinella, A.; Sodano, G., in Ref. 23.
29. Bruno, I.; Minale, L.; Pizza, C.; Zollo, F.; Riccio, R.; Mellon, F.A., *J. Chem. Soc., Perkin Trans. I*, 1984, 1875.
30. De Simone, F.; Dini, A.; Finamore, E.; Minale, L.; Pizza, C.; Riccio, R.; Zollo, F., *J. Chem. Soc., Perkin Trans. I*, 1981, 1855.

31. Riccio, R.; Minale, L.; Pizza, C.; Zollo, F.; Pusset, J., *Tetrahedron Lett.*, 1982, *23*, 2899.
32. Minale, L.; Riccio, R.; Pizza, C.; Zollo, F., *Proceedings of the Naito International Symposium on Natural Products*, Tokyo, November 1984 (in press).
33. Shimizu, Y., *J. Nat. Prod.*, 1985, *48*, 223.

Richard E. Moore, Gregory M. L. Patterson
Department of Chemistry, University of Hawaii, Honolulu, Hawaii 96822, U.S.A.

Culturing of Microalgae for Pharmaceutical Products at the University of Hawaii

Prompted by a few reports in the scientific literature that extracts of certain blue-green algae from marine, terrestrial, and freshwater sources contain cytotoxins, carcinogens, and substances that stimulate the healing of wounds,[1] researchers from this laboratory carried out the first systematic search for new antineoplastic agents from blue-green algae in the mid 1970s. This initial investigation resulted in the discovery of antileukemia activity in several marine cyanophytes, in particular ones belonging to the family Oscillatoriaceae.[2] The major active compound in two field-collected marine specimens from Eniwetok Atoll in the Marshall Islands, namely *Lyngbya majuscula* and a mixture of two Oscillatoriaceae identified as *Schizothrix calcicola* and *Oscillatoria nigroviridis*, was shown to be debromoaplysiatoxin, a highly inflammatory substance which had been isolated previously from the digestive tract of the sea hare *Stylocheilus longicauda*,[3] a gastoropod mollusk that feeds preferentially on *L. majuscula*.[4] Interestingly, in another study carried out in this laboratory a completely different antineoplastic agent, lyngbyatoxin A, was isolated from a variety of *L. majuscula* found at Kahala Beach on the island of Oahu.[5]

Debromoaplysiatoxin and lyngbyatoxin A, however, were only marginally active as antineoplastic agents. Both compounds were found to be potent tumor promoters.[6,7] Nevertheless, we were encouraged by the discovery of novel antineoplastic agents in *L. majuscula* and other marine Oscillatoriaceae. Specimens of blue-green algae were therefore collected from other islands in the subtropical and tropical Pacific basin for antineoplastic evaluation. Of 35 specimens that were found in Palau (Western Caroline Islands), Fanning Island (Line Islands), Johnston Island, and Molokai (Hawaii), five samples gave extracts that exhibited T/C ratios >200% in the murine P-388 lymphocytic leukemia test.[8] In contrast to our success in isolating the antineoplastic agents in *L. majuscula* and other Oscillatoriaceae, attempts to isolate the active principles from the five cyanophytes mentioned above were largely unsuccessful. *L. majuscula* was always one of the most abundant seaweeds on the pinnacles in Eniwetok Atoll lagoon and on the reefs around Oahu; other marine cyanophytes, however, were generally not found in large amounts in the field. The five blue-green algae could be collected in quantities sufficient only for initial screening, and all attempts to recollect the active cyanophytes for isolation and identification work failed; the algal blooms had either disappeared or had become inactive.[9] For example, a *Phormidium* sp. (Oscillatoriaceae) had been collected at Pohakuloa, Molokai, in November, 1977, and the crude methanolic extract of this cyanophyte had shown a T/C value of 210 at a dose of 12 mg/kg in the P-388 test with no signs of chronic toxicity and had completely cured Ehrlich ascites (EA) tumor in mice at a dose of 10 mg/kg. This *Phormidium* sp., however, was never found again; all of the *Phormidium* samples collected from the same area after November, 1977, were inactive. Similarly, in August, 1977, an *Oscillatoria* sp. had been collected from the reef in Arumizu Bay, Palau. The crude aqueous ethanolic extract of this blue-green alga had shown a T/C value of 205% at a dose of 5 mg/kg in the P-388 screen, again with no signs of chronic toxicity, and had completely cured EA at 4 mg/kg. When this *Oscillatoria* sp. was recollected at the same site in Palau two years later, the extract showed no antineoplastic activity.[9,10]

In addition to debromoaplysiatoxin, the abundant deep-water variety of *L. majuscula* in Eniwetok Atoll lagoon contained another marginally active antineoplastic agent, majusculamide C.[9,11] Further testing of this novel cyclic depsipeptide, however, revealed that it was a potent fungicide and quite effective against several economically important fungal plant pathogens such as *Phytophthora infestans*, the causative organism of tomato late blight, and *Plasmopora viticola*, the causative organism of grape downy mildew. Furthermore, majusculamide C was effective against strains of fungi that had become resistant to Ridomil, a currently used fungicide. The antifungal properties suggested that majusculamide C might have potential commercial value. Large quantities of the fungicide, however, were now needed for more advanced testing. Unfortunately, the logistics of collecting very large amounts of the cyanophyte at Eniwetok were unfavorable. Subsequent searches for majusculamide C-producing *L. majuscula* in other parts of the tropical Pacific were unsuccessful. To date we have found this variety of *L. majuscula* only on the pinnacles in the lagoon of Eniwetok Atoll.

To overcome the problems associated with field collections, we began a modest program in early 1981 to grow blue-green algae in the laboratory under carefully controlled conditions. From the onset we decided not to restrict ourselves to marine species, as there was no reason to believe that new pharmaceuticals and agrochemicals could not be found in freshwater and terrestrial blue-green algae. Besides, many freshwater and terrestrial blue-green algae are halotolerant and are probably found in the marine environment, and, conversely, many marine cyanophytes can adjust to freshwater environments.[12] Several natural products that are found in marine cyanophytes could, therefore, be present in freshwater and terrestrial species. For example, the toxins in dermatitis- and diarrhea-producing blue-green algae found in freshwater lakes and drinking-water reservoirs may be debromoaplysiatoxin- and lyngbyatoxin-type compounds.[13]

So far we have prepared over 300 unialgal cultures of blue-green algae and have tested extracts of most of these cyanophytes for cytotoxicity (KB), antineoplastic activity (P-388 lymphocytic leukemia in mice), and tumor-promoting and anti-tumor-promoting activity (HL-60 cell adhesion assay). This program has been fairly successful. About 2% of the extracts show consistent cytotoxic or antineoplastic activity and approximately 1% exhibit tumor-promoting or anti-tumor-promoting activity. Although our discovery rate for cytotoxicity and/or antineoplastic activity in extracts of cultured blue-green algae has not been as high as our 15% discovery rate in extracts of field-collected cyanophytes, we are very confident that at least 2% of the extracts of new isolates of cultured cyanophytes will show activity in these screens. Our conservative 2% discovery rate is somewhat lower than the 2.9% discovery rate of antineoplastic antibiotics in NCI's fermentation program.[14] In recent years, however, fermentation programs, especially in industry, have been so intense that the rediscovery rate of known cytotoxins and antineoplastic agents is frequently over 95%, as it is currently with cultured actinomycetes.[15] Algal cultivation programs should provide a greater rate of return as the algae have been relatively unexploited as sources of new pharmaceuticals.

In our program, algal material is obtained from a variety of worldwide freshwater, terrestrial, and marine environments. Most of our collections to date have been made in

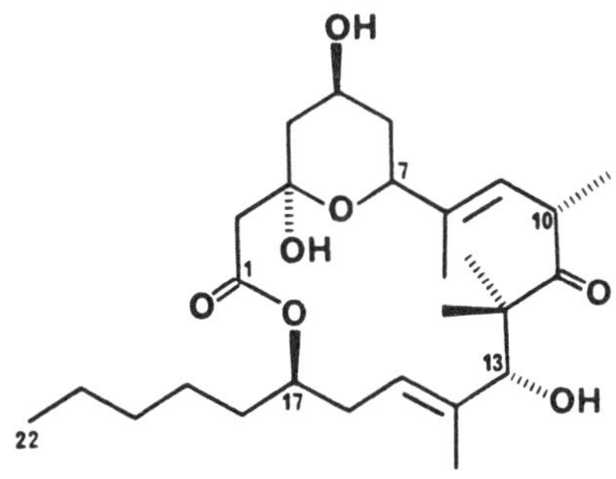

acutiphycin

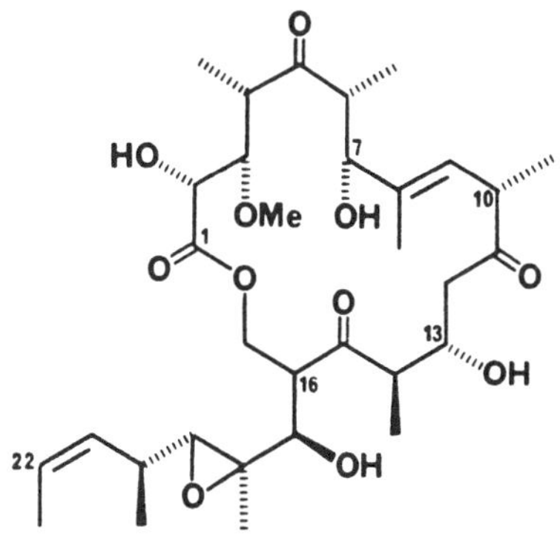

tedanolide

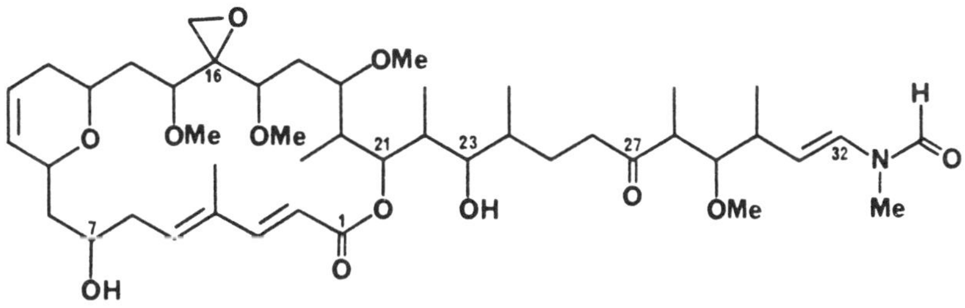

scytophycin B

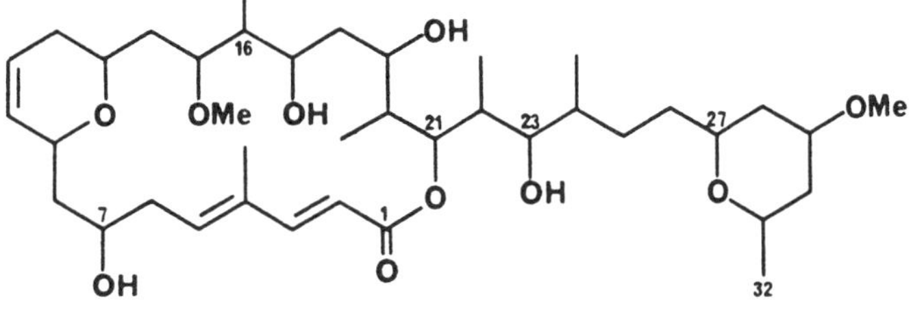

swinholide A

the subtropical and tropical regions of the Pacific basin. Initially an aliquot of the sample from the field is placed in a liquid medium which is formulated to enhance the growth of cyanophytes while generally retarding the growth of fungi, bacteria, and other groups of algae.[16] The medium contains nitrate as the sole nitrogen source, but no organic carbon source, and may contain cycloheximide to suppress eukaryotic cell growth. Media for marine isolates are supplemented with vitamins, especially B_{12}, which some marine blue-green algae have been shown to require.[17] After incubation, a portion of the growing algal material is removed and homogenized. Dilutions of this suspension are then spread, using a bent glass rod, on the surface of solidified media in Petri plates. After incubation for two to four weeks, algal colonies or filaments, free from other algal contaminants, are removed by the use of a wire needle or loop and streaked onto the surface of a second Petri dish. After sufficient sequential streak isolations have been made in this manner to yield algal clones free from other algae or fungi, cultures are transferred to liquid medium (initially 10 mL in culture tubes). These small volume cultures provide the inocula for subsequent scale-up.

Each isolate is grown in a 10-L culture to provide sufficient algal material for bioactivity screening. Should a positive result be obtained and subsequently confirmed with a second 10-L batch culture, 25-L batch cultures are then grown under the same conditions to provide sufficient material for chemical and biological characterization. About 20% of the 10-L batch cultures that show cytotoxicity or antineoplactic activity in the initial screen prove to be inactive on subsequent regrowth. Some of the confirmed actives lose activity for unknown reasons when subsequently grown in 25-L batch cultures and even again in 10-L cultures. For example, the crude extract of one of our isolates, identified as *Lyngbya limnetica*, showed high cytotoxicity against NIH3T3 cells ($ED_{50} <$ 8 μg/mL) in the initial screen, which was confirmed on regrowth of the alga. A few months later when the alga was regrown in 10- or 25-L batches to initiate isolation and identification studies, the extracts of the regrown alga showed no activity.

Roughly 0.5 g of freeze-dried alga is produced per liter of culture after an average 3-week incubation period. The 5 g of dried cells from a 10-L batch provides sufficient 30% ethanol extract for a wide variety of *in vitro* pharmacological screens. In addition to cytotoxins and antineoplastic agents, we have found that blue-green algae are excellent sources for new fungicides. About 3% of our cultured cyanophytes exhibit potent antimycotic activity.

To date our cultivation program has led to the discovery of the acutiphycins,[18] unusual macrolides from *Oscillatoria acutissima* having antineoplastic activity; the hapalindoles,[19] novel indole alkaloids from *Hapalosiphon fontinalis* having algicidal and fungicidal activity; and the scytophycins,[20] novel macrolides from *Scytonema pseudohofmanni* having potent cytotoxic and antifungal activity. It has also resulted in the identification of tubercidin, a previously know antitumor antibiotic, as the active antineoplastic agent and fungicide in *Tolypothrix byssoidea*.[21] The acutiphycins appear to be biogenetically related to tedanolide, a potent cytotoxin that has been isolated from the marine sponge *Tedania ignis*.[22] This is interesting since many marine natural products chemists have speculated that some secondary metabolites of sponges and tunicates result from microalgal symbionts. So far we feel that the scytophycins provide the strongest circumstantial evidence that symbiotic blue-green algae may play an important role in the production of some marine animal metabolites. The scytophycins are structurally very similar to swinholide A,[23] an antifungal agent from the Red Sea sponge *Theonella swinhoei*. Interestingly, a unicellular blue-green alga has been shown to be associated symbiotically with *T. swinhoei* from the Red Sea.[24]

The hapalindoles and the scytophycins may have commercial value. If these substances are going to reach the market place, large amounts of the hapalindoles and the scytophycins will have to be made available to industry for research and development. This means that large-scale cultivation equipment will have to be constructed to grow huge quantities of the blue-green algae that produce these compounds. Until the first commercially successful pharmaceutical or agrochemical from a blue-green alga is found, the chemical industry will be reluctant to invest a large amount of capital in large-scale cultivation facilities. In our laboratory we can only cultivate cyanophytes in open, indoor tanks of 175-L capacity. With these tanks we have been able to grow a few kilograms of *Hapalosiphon fontinalis* to supply the pharmaceutical industry with tens of grams of hapalindole A for some *in vivo* testing and structure-activity studies. These amounts are insufficient, however, as hundreds of grams will be needed for more advanced testing and evaluation.

In the last few years several new biotechnology companies have been formed that are dedicated to large-scale cultivation of microalgae for the production of specialty chemicals. One such company is Cyanotech, which recently began operation of a 4.1-acre experimental outdoor culture facility on the Big Island of Hawaii at Keahole Point, Kona. Arrangements are being made with Cyanotech to grow huge quantities of *Hapalosiphon fontinalis*. In the one experiment that has been conducted so far, *H. fontinalis* has been successfully grown in an open 500-L outdoor, raceway-style tank.

Very little work has been done in our laboratory on selecting strains and determining the optimum culture conditions for maximum production of hapalindoles and scytophycins. The concentrations of major nutrients and harvest time, however, are frequently important in maximizing secondary metabolite production. For example, production of the acutiphycins in *Oscillatoria acutissima* is highest when nitrate and phosphate are present in limiting or near-limiting amounts; the drug yields are drastically reduced when the concentration of either nutrient is increased. Addition of organic carbon or nitrogen sources to the mineral medium likewise decreases acutiphycin production. The acutiphycin yield is at a maximum when the alga is harvested after 3 weeks. At this point the culture is in the stationary phase of growth. A lower yield of acutiphycins is obtained if the harvest time is carried into the late stages of the stationary phase.

Acknowledgments. Our work on cultured blue-green algae is being supported by grants from the National Science Foundation (CHE83-03996) and the National Cancer Institute (CA12623-12).

REFERENCES

1. Baslow, M.H., "Marine Pharmacology", Krieger Publishing, Huntington, 1977.
2. Mynderse, J.S.; Moore, R.E.; Kashiwagi, M.; Norton, T.R., *Science Washington, D.C.)*, 1977, *196*, 538.
3. Kato, Y.; Scheuer, P.J., *Pure Appl. Chem.*, 1975, *41*, 1.
4. Switzer-Dunlap, M.; Hadfield, M., *J. Exp. Mar. Biol. Ecol.*, 1977, *29*, 245.
5. Cardellina II, J.H.; Marner, F.J.; Moore, R.E., *Science (Washington, D.C.)*, 1979, *294*, 193.
6. Fujiki, H.; Suganuma, M.; Hakii, H.; Bartolini, G.; Moore, R.E..; Takayama, S.; Sugimura, T., *J. Cancer Res. Clin. Oncol.*, 1984, *108*, 174.
7. Fujiki, H.; Suganuma, M.; Tahira, T.; Yoshioka, A.; Nakayasu, M.; Endo, Y.; Shudo, K.; Takayama, S.; Moore, R.E.; Sugimura, T., in "Cellular Interactions by Environmental Tumor Promoters", Fujiki, H., Hecker, E., Moore, R.E., Sugimura, T., Weinstein, I,B., Eds., Japan Scientific Societies Press, Tokyo, Japan, 1984, pp 37-45.
8. Kashiwagi, M.; Mynderse, J.S.; Moore, R.E.; Norton, T.R., *J. Pharm. Sci.*, 1980, *69*, 735.
9. Moore, R.E., *Pure Appl. Chem.*, 1982, *54*, 1919.

10. Patterson, G.M.L.; Norton, T.R.; Furusawa, E.; Furusawa, S.; Kashiwagi, M.; Moore, R.E., *Bot. Mar.*, 1984, *27*, 485.
11. Carter, D.C.; Moore, R.E.; Mynderse, J.S.; Niemczura, W.P.; Todd, J.S., *J. Org. Chem.*, 1984, *49*, 236.
12. Waterbury, J.B.; Stanier, R.Y., in "The Prokaryotes", Starr, M.P., Stolp, H., Truper, H.G., Balows, A., Schlegel, H.G., Eds., Springer Verlag, New York, 1981, pp 221-223.
13. Carmichael, W.W.; Moore, R.E.; Patterson, G.M.L., unpublished observations.
14. Douros, J.; Suffness, M., in "New Anticancer Drugs. Recent Results in Cancer Research", Carter, S.K., Sakurai, Y., Eds., Springer Verlag, New York, 1980, Vol. 70, pp 21-44.
15. Bradner, W.T., in "Cancer and Chemotherapy", Crooke, S.T., Prestayko, A.W., Eds., Academic Press, New York, 1980, Vol. I, pp 313-324.
16. Allen, M.M.; Stanier, R.Y., *J. Gen. Microbiol.*, 1968, *51*, 203.
17. Pintner, I.J.; Provasoli, L., *J. Gen. Microbiol.*, 1958, *18*, 190.
18. Barchi, J.J., Jr.; Moore, R.E.; Patterson, G.M.L., *J. Am. Chem. Soc.*, 1984, *106*, 8193.
19. Moore, R.E.; Cheuk, C.; Patterson, G.M.L., *J. Am. Chem. Soc.*, 1984, *106*, 6456.
20. Moore, R.E.; Patterson, G.M.L.; Mynderse, J.S.; Barchi, J., Jr.; Norton, T.R.; Furusawa, E.; Furusawa, S., *Pure Appl. Chem.*, 1986, *58*, 263.
21. Barchi, J.J., Jr.; Norton, T.R.; Furusawa, E.; Patterson, G.M.L.; Moore, R.E., *Phytochemistry*, 1983, *22*, 2851.
22. Schmitz, F.J.; Gunasekera, S.P.; Yalamanchili, G.; Hossain, M.B.; van der Helm, D., *J. Am. Chem. Soc.*, 1984, *106*, 7251.
23. Carmely, S.; Kashman, Y., *Tetrahedron Lett.* 1985, *25*, 511.
24. Wilkinson, C.R., in "Biologie des Spongiaires", Levi, C., Boury-Esnault, N., Eds., Centre National de la Recherche Scientifique, Paris, France, 1979, pp 373-380.

Lantz S. Crawley
American Cyanamid Company, Agricultural Research Division, Princeton, New Jersey 08540, U.S.A.

The Search for New Products for Agriculture from Marine Sources by American Cyanamid

American Cyanamid is a research-based biotechnology and chemical company with its headquarters in Wayne, New Jersey. The company develops, manufactures, and markets proprietary medical, agricultural, chemical, and consumer products around the world. At a 640-acre agricultural research center located in Princeton, New Jersey, just four miles from the campus of Princeton University, research is conducted to support existing business and to develop new agents for use in agriculture world-wide.

Research is divided into two main areas--plant and animal. In the plant area there are basic programs in herbicides, insecticides, fungicides, plant growth regulators, and in plant molecular biology. In the animal area novel agents to improve animal growth and production are being sought, and work is also being done in nutrition and physiology, chemotherapy and immunology, and molecular biology.

A key element of our research strategy is the development of unique high-capacity screens for broad evaluation of compounds from diverse sources. These include compounds synthesized by chemists at Princeton or other Cyanamid research locations as well as compounds obtained from other industrial or university investigators. We also actively evaluate soil fermentation samples and natural products isolated from terrestrial sources. Today I would like to discuss our approach to screening and some of our recent work in three areas--insecticides, herbicides, and partitioning agents (compounds which decrease the fat and increase the lean meat in animals). I hope by this means to give you a better understanding of our keen interest in evaluating natural products from marine sources.

The world insecticide market is estimated at over four and one-half billion dollars. Natural products have long been a source of new leads and often serve as models for chemical synthesis. Well-known examples of natural products employed directly as insecticides include nicotine, rotenone, the pyrethrins, and, more recently, azadirachtin. Examples of insecticides based on natural products (Figure 1) include the carbamates (*e.g.*, Furadan® 1), pyrethroids (*e.g.*, Pay-Off® 2) and dimethylamino dithiolanes (*e.g.*, Paydan® 3).

With the exception of 3, these insecticides were derived from terrestrial plants. The traditional medicinal use and the greater accessibility of terrestrial natural products have made them the initial source of materials for evaluation as insecticides. The wealth of novel insecticidal chemistry still to be learned from terrestrial sources is exemplified by

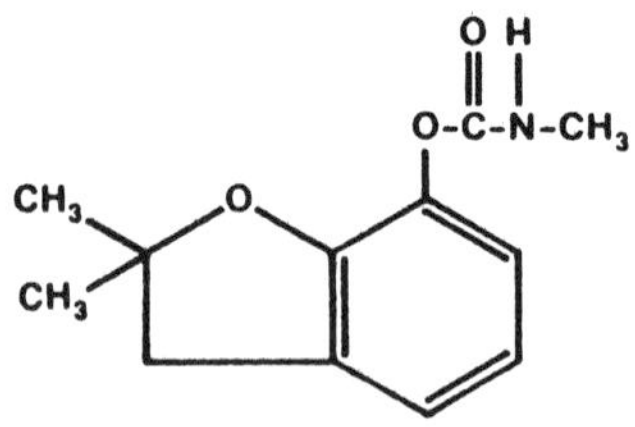

1 FURADAN®

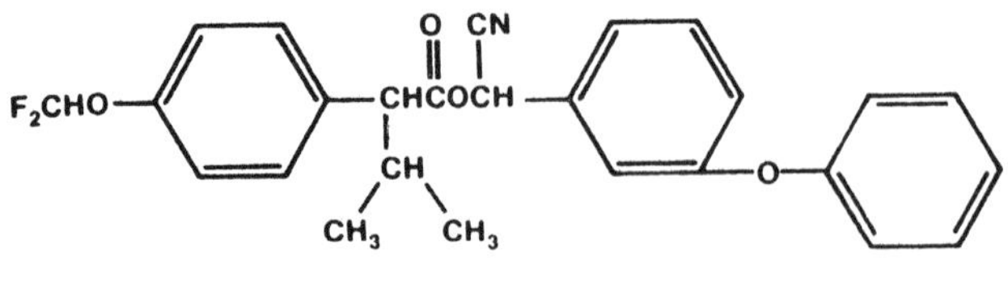

2 PAY-OFF®

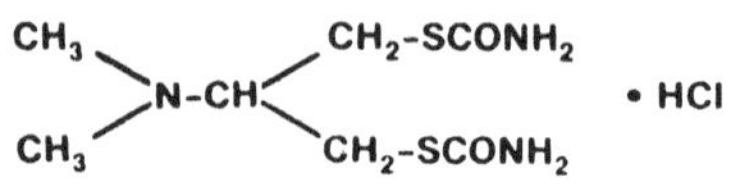

3 PAYDAN®

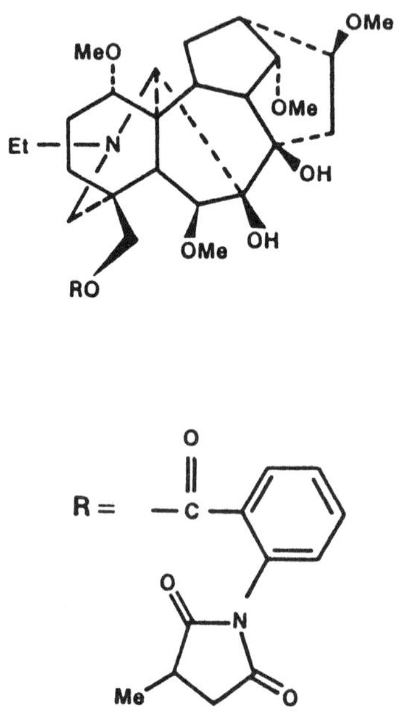

Methyllycaconitine (4)

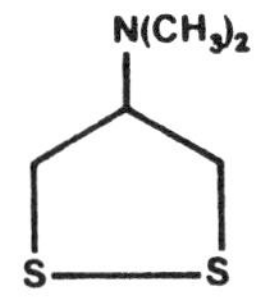

5 Nereistoxin

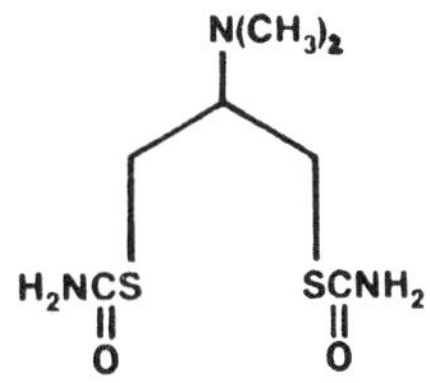

6 Cartap

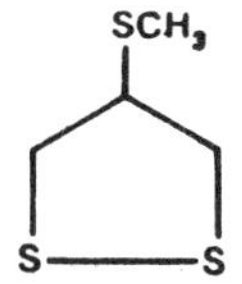

7 Charatoxin

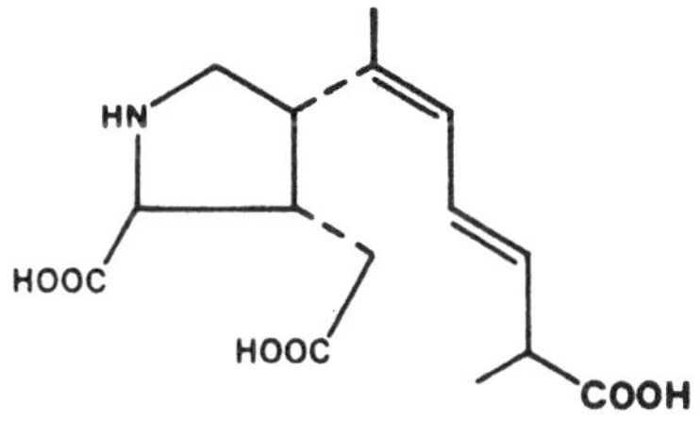

8 Domoic Acid

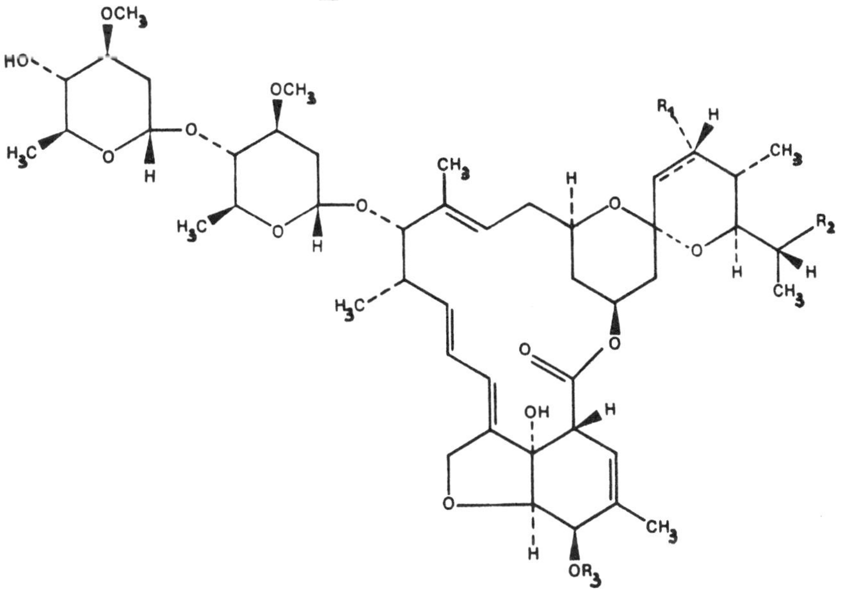

9 Avermectins

the recent isolation in our laboratories of an alkaloid (Figure 2), methyllycaconitine (4), from *Delphinium* seeds;[1] it has potent cholinergic and insecticidal activities.

Only recently has our attention turned to the ocean as a source of new insecticidal materials. A number of marine natural products are known to be potent toxins and the few that have been characterized, such as tetrodotoxin and saxitoxin, have proved to be valuable tools for the pharmacologist.[2] Nereistoxin (5), isolated by Nitta in 1934 from the marine annelid *Lumbriconereis heteropoda* Marenz, which is commonly used as fishing bait in Japan, was shown to be 4-(N,N-dimethylamino)-1,2-dithiolane by Okaichi and Hashimoto.[3] A synthetic analogue of this material, cartap (Padan® 6), a major rice insecticide in Japan, is especially effective against the rice stemborer. A related toxin, charatoxin (7), from the marine alga *Chara globularis* Thuillier[4], has recently been identified and shown to be insecticidal by researchers at Cheminova.[5]

Both nereistoxin[6] and charatoxin[7] appear to exert their toxic effects at the cholinergic synapse in insects, a nervous system target. They block cholinergic neurotransmission by inhibiting receptor and/or ion channel function. The physiological effect of these toxins on insects consists of rapid onset of paralysis, followed by death.

Because of the apparent abundance of insecticidal products from natural sources, American Cyanamid has expanded its program to evaluate both terrestrial- and marine-derived natural products as potential insecticides. In addition to direct screening on insects, which is the primary focus of our screening operation in Princeton, active materials can be evaluated for bioactivity on the insect nerve and muscle systems. Included in this neurobiological screening operation is the cholinergic nervous system in the insect. This activity is evaluated by neurochemical receptor binding studies on nicotinic and muscarinic sites and by neurophysiological assays. The *Delphinium* alkaloid methyllycaconitine (4) was shown to be the most potent inhibitor of the nicotinic acetylcholine receptor in insects yet identified, being more potent than the snake toxin alpha-bungarotoxin.

Other neurotoxin target sites that can be evaluated in the laboratory include the glutamate (excitatory) and GABA (inhibitory) synapses on invertebrate muscle. These target sites are known to be important in the mode of action of two naturally occurring insecticidal materials, domoic acid (8), a potent glutamate agonist derived from the marine alga *Chondria armata*,[8,9] and avermectin (9), derived from a soil streptomycete,[10] which appears to act on the GABA system in insects.[11] Other nervous system target sites that are evaluated in insecticide research include ion channels such as the sodium channel, the site of action of DDT and the pyrethroids, as well as the marine neurotoxins tetrodotoxin and saxitoxin.

For cholinergic assays, receptor binding using radio-labeled bungarotoxin can be used to evaluate nicotinic agonist/antagonist activity and physiological experiments can be conducted on the *Periplaneta americana* cercal nerve preparation, a nicotinic cholinergic synapse. Similarly, radio-labeled quinuclidinyl benzilate can be utilized as a radio-ligand for the study of muscarinic receptor function in insects. Glutamate function can be assayed in a *P. americana* hindgut preparation formed with insect saline in an organ bath. This type of assay is similar to the guinea pig ileum assay used widely in the pharmaceutical industry. GABA activity can be assayed on a number of invertebrate muscle systems, including those of crustacea.

Another potentially important mode of action of natural product insecticides is disruption of biogenic amine function. Crustaceans, insects, and mammals all utilize amines as transmitters and modulators in nerve and muscle function. In insects those amines include dopamine (10), octopamine (11), and serotonin (12). Many terrestrial plants elaborate simple amine-related compounds that may have pestistatic properties in the natural

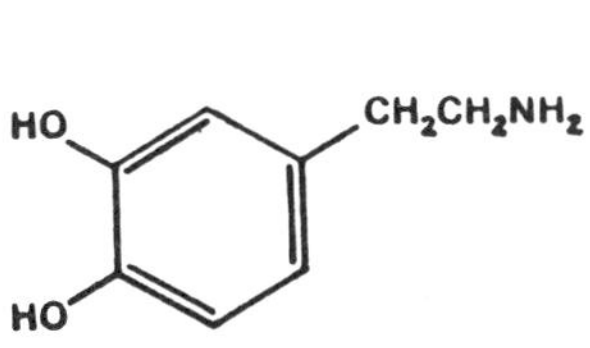

10 **Dopamine**

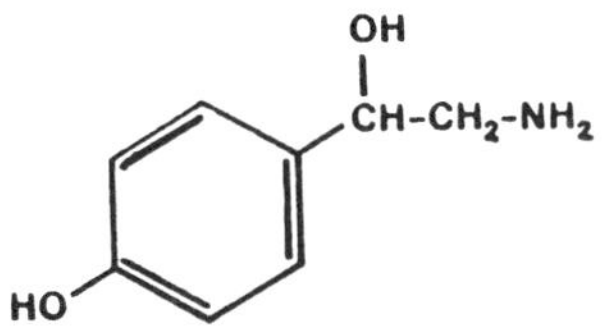

11 **Octopamine**

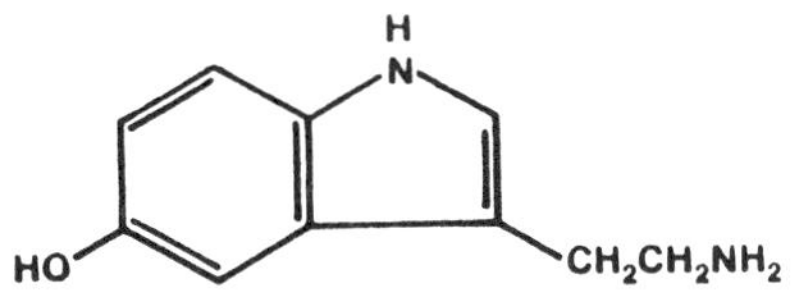

12 **Serotonin**

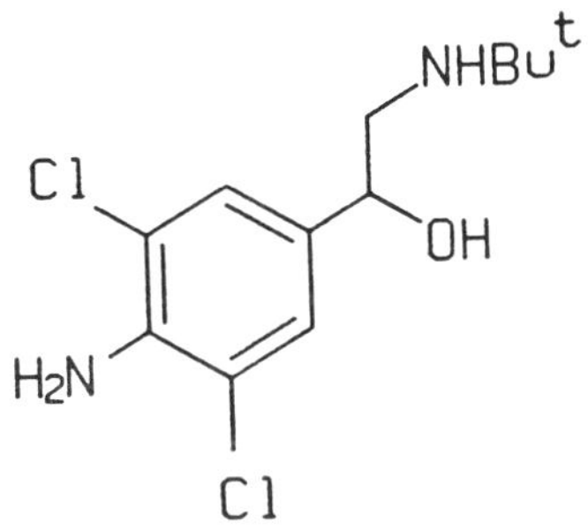

13

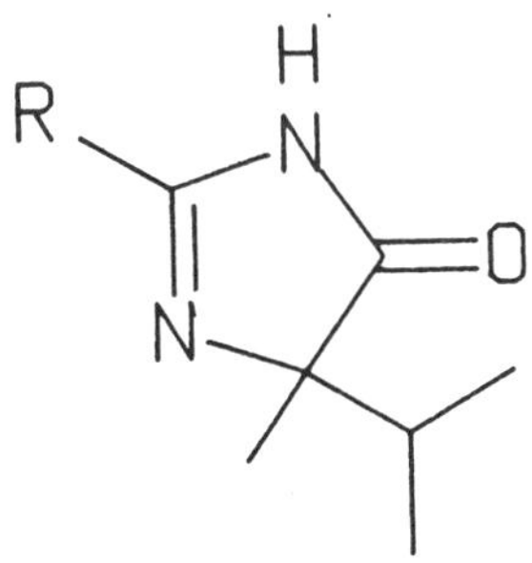

R =

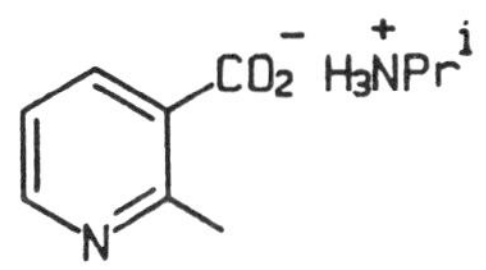

14

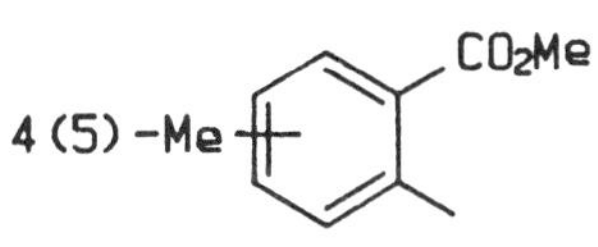

15

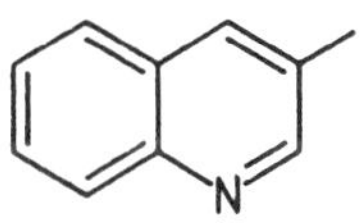

16

environment. I anticipate that marine sources will also be rich in amine-related chemistry.

Such biogenic amines will also be of interest in the new area of animal research called "partitioning agents". In 1984 researchers in our laboratory reported that clenbuterol (13), a commercial bronchial dilator, was capable not only of stimulating growth of meat-producing animals and improving conversion of feedstuffs to edible tissue, but also of favorably altering the composition of the carcass by increasing accretion of muscle and limiting fat deposition.[12-15] Clenbuterol has a dramatic effect on carcass composites in lambs. There is increased muscling, especially in the leg/rump area, and the cut at the twelfth rib shows a greater cross sectional area of rib muscle and a corresponding decrease in subcutaneous fat depth. A similar effect can be obtained with this or a number of related agents in broilers, swine, and cattle.

Several assay systems have been developed to screen for compounds with such activity and to conduct initial evaluations. For *in vivo* primary screening we use a mouse growth assay in which the growth-promoting and fat-lowering properties of compounds are compared to control and known active compounds. Active compounds are further evaluated *in vivo* in a chick growth assay and performance trials in target species such as broilers, swine, lambs and cattle. We have also developed a proprietary screen to determine the effect of selected compounds on various pathways of lipid metabolism. This system has been adapted to allow rapid screening of natural products from terrestrial or marine sources and evaluation of soil fermentation products. I have no estimate of the market potential of such agents, it is expected, however, to be considerable.

The herbicide market is one of the largest in the agricultural industry and is estimated at close to six billion dollars. Cyanamid has recently discovered and developed a new class of herbicides called the imidazolinones.[16] Three products--arsenal (14), a total vegetation control agent; assert (15), a cereal herbicide which is used on wild oats and blackgrass problems in wheat; and scepter (16) for the control of a broad spectrum of weeds in soybeans--are ready for commercialization.

Work in our laboratory[17] and in collaboration with MGI, a genetic engineering firm, showed that the mechanism of action of these herbicides involved the inhibition of acetohydroxyacid synthase (AHAS), the first common enzyme in the biosynthetic pathway of the essential amino acids leucine, isoleucine, and valine. To exploit this finding we developed a microtiterplate assay for rapid screening of additional compounds for their ability to inhibit the AHAS enzyme. Since we began the screen, we have identified several new chemical classes that will inhibit this enzyme, and we are trying to develop similar assays for other enzymes involved in critical biochemical pathways in plants.

To summarize, we have a number of *in vitro* and *in vivo* screens to evaluate compounds from diverse sources rapidly. In the past this approach has resulted in new products, or compounds that became products through semi-synthetic modification. Additionally, novel agents detected in these screens often function as models for our synthesis programs or serve as probes for increasing our understanding of biochemical mechanisms in plants and animals.

Lastly, we believe that the Harbor Branch/SeaPharm project will provide a unique source of bioactive compounds that should find significant application in the agricultural industry.

REFERENCES

1. Jennings, K.R.; Brown, D.B.; Wright, D.P., "Methyllycaconitine, a Naturally Occurring Insecticide With a High Affinity for the Insect Cholinergic Receptor (submitted for publication).
2. Hashimoto, Y., "Marine Toxins and Other Bioactive Marine Metabolites", Japan Sci. Press, Tokyo, 1979.
3. Okaichi, T.; Hashimoto, Y., *Bull. Jpn. Soc. Sci. Fish.*, 1962, *28*, 93; *Agric. Biol. Chem.*, 1962, *26*, 224.
4. Anthoni, V.; Christophersen, C.; Madsen, J.O.; Wium-Andersen, S.; Jacobsen, N., *Phytochemistry*, 1980, *19*, 1228.
5. Jacobsen, N.; Pedersen, L.E.K., *Pest. Sci.*, 1983, *24*, 90.
6. Narahashi, T., in "Marine Pharmacognosy", D. Martin & G. Padilla, Eds., Academic Press, New York, 1973.
7. Nielson, L.E.; Pedersen, L.E.K., *Experientia*, 1984, *40*, 186.
8. Maeda, M.; Kodama, T.; Tanaka, T.; Ohfune, Y.; Nomoto, K.; Nishimura, K.; Fjuita, T.J., *Pest. Sci.*, 1984, *9*, 27.
9. Castle, F.; Evans, R.H.; Kirkpatrick, J.N.P., *Comp. Biochem. Physiol.*, 1984, *77C*, 399.
10. Putter, I.; MacConnell, J.G.; Preiser, F.A.; Haidri, A.A.; Ristich, S.S.; Dybas, R.A., *Experientia*, 1981, *37*, 963.
11. Fritz, L.C.; Wang, C.C.; Gorio, A., *Proc. Natl. Acad. Sci. USA*, 1979, *76*, 2062.
12. Asato, G.; Baker, P.K.; Bass, R.T.; Bentley, T.J.; Chari, S.; Dalrymple, R.H.; France, D.J.; Gingher, P.E.; Lences, B.L.; Pascavage, J.J.; Pensack, J.M.; Ricks, C.A., *Agric. Biol. Chem.*, 1984, *48*, 2883.
13. Baker, P.K.; Dalrymple, R.H.; Ingle, D.L.; Ricks, C.A., *J. Animal Sci.*, 1984, *59*, 1256.
14. Dalrymple, R.H.; Baker, P.K.; Gingher, P.E.; Ingle, D.L.; Pensack, J.M.; Ricks, C.A., *Poultry Sci.*, 1984, *63*, 2376.
15. Ricks, C.A.; Dalrymple, R.H.; Baker, P.K.; Ingle, D.L., *J. Animal Sci.*, 1984, *59*, 1247.
16. Los, M., *ACS Symposium Series*, 1984, *255*, 29.
17. Shaner, D.L.; Anderson, P.C.; Stidham, M.A., *Plant Physiol.*, 1984, *76*, 545.

Juan Carlos Torres
SeaPharm, Inc., 791 Alexander Road, Princeton, New Jersey 08540, U.S.A.

SeaPharm's Approach to Marine Pharmaceutical Research

SEAPHARM

SeaPharm is a young biotechnology company, formed in 1983, engaged in pharmaceutical research aimed at the development of new therapeutic agents derived from marine plants and animals. SeaPharm's head office is in Princeton, New Jersey, but its laboratories are located in Fort Pierce, Florida, where it is associated with the Harbor Branch Foundation (HBF),* an oceanographic research institution at which many superb underwater research tools have been developed. The equipment maintained at the Harbor Branch Foundation allows a thorough and wide-ranging exploration of the marine environment.

SeaPharm occupied a temporary laboratory at Harbor Branch in 1984 and moved into its permanent laboratory there in 1985. It presently employs about 30 scientists--half chemists, half biologists. Early funding of the company has been derived from HBF, venture capital, and contracts with government and industrial sources.

RATIONALE FOR A MARINE PHARMACEUTICAL SEARCH

The decision to search for pharmaceuticals from marine species is really based on two observations. One is that natural products are good sources of drugs; natural products obtained from terrestrial sources account for 47% of the drugs developed for human consumption. The other observation is that, just as most of the earth's surface is covered by water, so, too, do 80% of the earth's animal species live in the sea. A rich source, a potential pharmacopoeia of new drugs, remains relatively untapped.

A useful analogy, which I believe is relevant to the theme of these talks and to the renewed resolve to study "pharmaceuticals and the sea", can be drawn between two very different businesses--the oil industry and the pharmaceutical industry. Oil is, after all, a natural product, and in the early days of oil exploration almost all discoveries were made on-shore. As seismic exploration, off-shore drilling, and other advanced technologies came into use, most discoveries arose from off-shore sources. We believe that the state of the pharmaceutical industry today is similar in many ways to that of the oil industry 20-25 years ago.

---

* Now the Harbor Branch Oceanographic Institution (eds.)

It must, of course, be pointed out that the search for marine pharmaceuticals is not entirely new. As described in other sections of this volume, there have been some successes, especially with compounds based on marine natural product models. Moreover, some pharmaceutical products of marine origin are already familiar (*i.e.*, cod liver oil, agar, carageenan and some cardiovascular and antitumor agents and muscle relaxants of minor importance), and a number of marine-derived products have important market value. Cephalosporins, which are among the most sophisticated antibiotics, with annual sales of almost $1 billion, are based on studies of a Mediterranean marine microorganism.

FOCUS OF RESEARCH

Analysis of pharmaceutical sales figures confirms the existence of a good number of effective drugs in some areas--antibiotics and analgesics, for example--but a notable lack of antitumor agents (especially drugs effective against slow-growing tumors), as well as antifungal, cardiotonic, and antiviral agents and drugs effective as immunostimulants or immunosuppressives. Drugs currently prescribed in these areas are often not very effective and have potentially fatal side effects, among them bone marrow depression, kidney failure, arrhythmia, and cardiac blockage. It is precisely in the field of antitumor and antiviral activity that marine natural products already show excellent promise. Research so far has indicated a greater number and variety of anticancer compounds in marine organisms than in terrestrial species. Moreover, marine microorganisms such as blue-green algae offer a higher percentage of antitumor compounds of novel structural types than do actinomycetes, fungi, and bacteria, the traditional land-based sources of antitumor agents. A vigorous effort to increase the volume of marine natural products research could, therefore, be most significant in meeting man's need for new drugs.

SEAPHARM EXPEDITIONS

As noted in Dr. Rinehart's section of this volume, the difficulties of collecting marine organisms and of classifying novel species have complicated the pharmaceutical evaluation of marine plants and animals. Recently, however, modern technology has been applied to underwater explorations to solve many of these problems and to allow routine and widespread collections at depths greater than 100 feet.

SeaPharm expeditions to locate bioactive marine species are carried out on board Harbor Branch vessels--the flagship *R/V Seward Johnson*, 175 feet in length; the *R/V Sea Diver*, 100 feet; and the *R/V Edwin Link*, 125 feet. Thus far, these expeditions have concentrated on the Bahamas, but an expedition is scheduled this month to the Western Caribbean (Belize, Honduras, Cayman Islands) and one in late 1986 to the Galapagos Islands. Both the *Seward Johnson* and the *Sea Diver* are equipped with laboratory space for bioassays, and all three vessels are equipped with the Johnson-Sea-Link (JSL) submersibles. These were designed by the late Edwin Link and developed by the Harbor Branch Foundation. The submersibles are purpose-built and have some special features.

The acrylic bubble of the JSL affords nearly 360° visibility, and the multifunctional robotic arm with jaw, clambucket, and suction devices permits the collection of almost any marine sample. A storage array of 12 buckets that rotate on a "lazy Susan" allows the separation and storage of individual samples during a dive.

The submersible is launched and recovered by means of an A-frame or crane that lifts it to and from its secured position on the deck of its mother ship. The *Seward Johnson* was designed to carry two submersibles, and its modern scientific laboratories can support 13 scientists. Its state-of-the-art tracking system allows scientists to return later to an exact collection site, on the surface or underwater, and provides for monitoring of the underwater submersible by the mother ship on the surface. The *Sea Diver*, although older and smaller, has similar facilities.

The marine samples collected by submersible, SCUBA, snorkeling, or inter-tidal techniques are taken immediately to the research vessel for sorting, labeling, identification, and photography. A small sample (*ca.* 2 g) of each organism is then ground, extracted, and bioassayed in the shipboard laboratories. Marine specimens are thus screened immediately after collection for biological activity, and the remainder of the sample is quickly frozen.

The bioassays used were described by Dr. Rinehart in his section of this volume. A plaque assay is used for judging antiviral activity (HSV-1, VSV), a cell-growth inhibition assay (P388 or L1210) for cytotoxicity, plate assays for antimicrobial activity (bacteria and fungi), and mitogen-stimulated assays (T-cell, B-cell) for immunomodulation. A total of 50 to 100 samples per day are usually collected and assayed. Larger amounts of interesting, bioactive samples are then re-collected at once, while the taxonomists present on the ship observe the organisms in their natural habitats.

ISOLATION AND IDENTIFICATION OF ACTIVE COMPOUNDS

Once the samples are returned to Fort Pierce, the active extracts are re-assayed; in case of negative results, the original frozen sample is re-extracted. Positive samples are then tested against traditional viruses, cell lines, fungi, etc. The next stage--*in vivo* testing--is presently carried out elsewhere, but animal facilities are under construction. Samples are also tested for additional bioactivities by other companies under contracts with SeaPharm.

The process of isolating bioactive materials from marine specimens, of separating and purifying the compounds responsible for that bioactivity, and of assigning chemical structures to compounds available in very small amounts is often time-consuming, difficult and has sometimes proved impossible. In some cases, bioactivity was observed long before structure elucidation was achieved.

However, recent improvements in spectroscopy and chromatography, some of which are described in the sections by Drs. Moore and Nakanishi, have made isolation and structure elucidation much easier. For example, the study of the antitumor marine depsipeptide, didemnin B, now in Phase I clinical trials, was hastened by advances in high-field nuclear magnetic resonance spectroscopy, high-resolution fast atom bombardment mass spectrometry, and high-performance liquid chromatography. There is another aspect of the rapid structural elucidation of didemnin B to be noted. Didemnin B was obtained in the relatively high yield of *ca.* 6.6 grams per 100 kilograms of the tunicate *Trididemnum sp.*[**] This can be contrasted with the 40 mg of bryostatin obtained per 100 kilograms of the Californian bryozoan *Bugula neritina.* In other cases still smaller amounts of the active materials are available. The difficulty in supplying adequate amounts of compounds for clinical trials or commercialization has long been regarded as a major hindrance to the development of marine pharmaceuticals. While the problem remains, there are solutions on the horizon. In favorable cases--abundant species, high concentration, exceedingly active compound--the compounds may be obtained from natural sources. In other cases, involving relatively simple molecules, the compounds can be synthesized on a commercial scale by skilled organic chemists. In the future, scarcities of bioactive marine-derived materials may be alleviated by aquaculture, by new tissue culture techniques, or by fermentation after genetic engineering. The latter

---

** Now identified as *T. solidum* (eds.)

quire the active collaboration of marine biologists and considerable basic research on the marine organisms involved.

EXTRAMURAL PROGRAM

In addition to carrying out research on-board HBF vessels and in laboratories at Fort Pierce, SeaPharm also maintains a number of collaborative research contracts with scientists at academic institutions throughout the world, but mainly in the Western Pacific--New Zealand, Australia, and Okinawa. These contracts enhance considerably the geographical scope of SeaPharm's collections and have provided some of the most active samples to date. Thus, New Zealand waters have yielded a very potent antiviral agent from a tunicate and a compound active against leukemia from a sponge.

CONCLUSIONS

As noted at the beginning of this section, SeaPharm is a new company. However, it is the largest company devoted to the marine pharmaceutical field. It operates with the advantage of close cooperation with a high-technology oceanographic institution. The extensive shipboard screening program has already provided a number of promising new leads in the antitumor and antiviral areas. Developing these and others to come should keep us busy for a number of years.

Section IV

Techniques for the Analysis and Isolation of Marine Natural Products

Richard E. Moore, Walter P. Niemczura
Department of Chemistry, University of Hawaii, Honolulu, Hawaii 96822, U.S.A.

New NMR Techniques for Structure Determination

The changes that have occurred in NMR in the first half of this decade have been astounding. Major improvements and discoveries were made in the 1970s in superconducting magnet technology, pulsed Fourier transform (FT) techniques and data processing, permitting natural products chemists to handle complex structure problems effectively for the first time. The early 1980s, however, brought the introduction of routine two-dimensional (2-D) NMR spectroscopy and with it a dramatic change in methodology for structure determination.

Jeener proposed the concept of 2-D FT-NMR spectroscopy in 1971, but it was not until 1976 that Ernst and co-workers described the detailed theoretical explanation of this revolutionary technique.[1] Their publication was quickly followed by an overwhelming number of papers describing a wide variety of experiments utilizing the 2-D approach. These experiments can all be characterized by their four-part structure (preparation, evolution, mixing, and detection), which contains a variable delay time (t_1) in the evolution period. Taken collectively, all 2-D experiments can be categorized broadly as one of three types: 1) chemical shift correlation spectroscopy, 2) J-spectroscopy, or 3) multiple quantum coherence spectroscopy.[2-4]

The first 2-D experiment, proposed by Jeener, was the homonuclear chemical shift correlation experiment. This very powerful alternative to homonuclear double resonance spectroscopy is familiar to all natural products chemists and is often referred to as the COSY experiment (COrrelation SpectroscopY) or HOMCOR. When combined with a heteronuclear (typically ^{1}H-^{13}C) chemical shift correlation spectrum (HETCOR or CSCM), it allows the structural chemist to solve fairly complex structures quickly with relatively small amounts of material.

COSY spectra are typically depicted as contour plot of square matrices. Each matrix contains a line of diagonal peaks connecting two opposing corners of the matrix. (A sideways projection of these diagonal peaks would appear identical to the standard one-dimensional spectrum.) Each matrix also contains cross peaks, which are not located on the diagonal line, but which line up with, or correlate, two points on the diagonal axis. These cross peaks, therefore, denote which resonances are spin coupled. In a conventional COSY spectrum cross peaks are generally much less intense than diagonal peaks and are frequently absent for weakly coupled spin-systems. Moreover, cross peaks are often either obscured by large peaks along the diagonal axis or sufficiently overlapped with other cross peaks that ambiguities arise in interpretation. Modifications of the

COSY experiment which circumvent these problems have been devised. One variation (SUPER COSY) uses a pulse scheme which removes the antiphase character of the multiplets of the cross peaks and introduces antiphase character into the multiplets of the diagonal peaks, resulting in an increase in the intensities of the cross peaks and a decrease in the intensities of the diagonal peaks.[5] In another variation--the delayed COSY experiment--fixed delays added to both the evolution and detection periods enhance magnetization transfer between protons that are weakly coupled. This results in cross peaks for weakly coupled protons having small coupling constants, but less intense cross peaks are then found for the more strongly coupled protons.[6] This experiment must frequently be repeated with different delay times in order to optimize visualization of the cross peaks due to small long-range couplings, but it provides the structural chemist with a way to connect proton spin systems that are separated by quaternary carbons or heteroatoms. Four-bond interglycosidic $^4J_{HCOCH}$ couplings can be detected by the delayed COSY method and are useful for sequencing small- to medium-sized oligosaccharides.[7] An improved version of the COSY experiment uses a double-quantum filter (DQF) essentially to remove uncoupled resonances along the diagonal;[8] this experiment is very useful for eliminating large solvent peaks such as that for water. The multiplet structure of cross peaks in the ω_1 dimension, the dimension created by the variable delays in the evolution period, are removed by ω_1-decoupling, which has also been used to obtain better resolution in the COSY spectrum.[2,9]

One of the major difficulties in solving gross structures of complex molecules by NMR spectroscopy is the problem of connecting proton spin systems that are separated by quaternary carbons or heteroatoms. Several elegant 2-D experiments have been designed to address this problem. In addition to the delayed COSY experiment, long range heteronuclear chemical shift correlation spectroscopy (long range HETCOR or CSCM), long range heteronuclear J resolved spectroscopy (LRJR)[10,11], 2D NOE spectroscopy (NOESY), and rotating-frame Overhauser spectroscopy (ROESY or CAMELSPIN)[12,13] are useful methods for sequencing partial structures through quaternary carbons or heteroatoms. Some one-dimensional experiments have also been devised to deal with this problem, for example, selective population inversion[14-16] and selective polarization transfer.[17]

In this paper we illustrate the use of a new 2-D experiment, namely homonuclear relayed coherence transfer (RCT) spectroscopy, to determine unambiguous connectivities in COSY spectra of macromolecules such as polypeptides, polysaccharides, and polyketides. Also presented is an example of a new one-dimensional experiment, namely selective polarization transfer (selective INEPT) spectroscopy, which is useful for connecting partial structures through quaternary carbons and heteroatoms.

HOMONUCLEAR RELAYED COHERENCE TRANSFER NMR SPECTROSCOPY

Unambiguous connectivities are obtained from a COSY spectrum only when all of the coupled protons have unique chemical shifts. In elucidating the structures of macromolecules, however, the higher incidence of superimposed chemical shifts limits the effectiveness of the conventional COSY experiment. For example, in identifying amino acid units in a cyclic polypeptide using the COSY method, one is frequently confronted with superimposed α-proton resonances which make it impossible to establish directly which set of resonances belongs to a particular amino acid residue. Generally, connectivities can be established between the amide NH and α-proton resonances, but α-proton chemical shift degeneracy prevents unambiguous connectivities between the amide NH and β-proton resonances. This problem is readily solved by the homonuclear relayed coherence transfer (RCT) experiment, which provides additional cross peaks between amide NH and β-proton resonances.

The RCT experiment utilizes the basic pulse sequence outlined by Eich *et al.*[18] and shown in Figure 1. The experiment starts with the usual generation of transverse magnetization and evolution period, but the mixing pulse, that is, the second 90° pulse in the normal COSY experiment, is replaced by one or more 90°-τ-180°-τ-90° "relay" steps, where each step passes information from indirectly spin-coupled protons to the observed proton. The single-relay experiment can be visualized as back-to-back COSY experiments. The first 90° pulse generates transverse magnetization, which is allowed to evolve for a variable period t_1. The second 90° pulse transfers magnetization between coupled spins, thus frequency-labeling each spin with information from its coupled partner. In the simple AMX spin system where $J_{AX}=0$, for example, spin A is labeled with M, spin M is labeled with A and X, and X is labeled with M, resulting in the mixed spins A+M, M+(A+X), and X+M. The spins are allowed to precess for a period $\tau=(4J)^{-1}$ at which time the 180° pulse causes the diverging spins to refocus at a time τ, thereby removing any added chemical shift modulation during this period. The final 90° pulse again passes spin information between each coupled pair, since each spin has been previously labeled, however, information is actually passed between coupled pairs of labeled spins. In the AMX spin system the labeled spin A+M receives information from the labeled spin M+(A+M) and so on. Acquisition of the FID at this point detects signals from A+(M+X), M+(A+X), and X+(A+M), thereby establishing the connectivities in the whole spin system.

The usefulness of the RCT experiment is illustrated in the following example. The conventional COSY16 spectrum of a tridecaacetate derivative of a novel α-cyclodextrin isolated from the cultured blue-green alga *Tolypothrix byssoidea*[19] is shown in Figure 2 (upper left corner). The signals for the methine protons in each of the six α-glucose unities in the molecule are readily discernible. For example, the squares indicate the connectivities for the protons on carbons 1-5 of sugar unit A. Note, however, that the positions of the two protons on C-6 can not be detected unambiguously. Even the use of other solvents for the COSY spectrum fails to reveal the chemical shifts of the C-6 protons. The RCT experiment, however, allows a ready solution to this problem. The RCT spectrum of the α-cyclodextrin tridecaacetate, shown in Figure 2 (upper right corner), reveals two additional cross peaks for the H-3 signal, one reflecting the coupling of H-2 to H-1 and the other the coupling of H-4 to H-5. Further inspection of the RCT spectrum shows that three additional off-diagonal peaks are present for the H-4 signal, one reflecting the coupling of H-3 to H-2 and the other the coupling of H-5 to the non-equivalent protons on C-6 of sugar unit A. The connectivities of the protons on C-5 and C-6 can also be obtained by the double relayed coherence transfer (RCT2) experiment. The RCT2 spectrum of the α-cyclodextrin tridecaacetate, depicted in Figure 2 (bottom left corner), shows cross peaks from the H-3 signal to both protons on C-6. The RCT and RCT2 experiments allow unambiguous assignments of all the chemical shifts for the C-6 protons on the six α-glucose units.

The relay experiments on the α-cyclodextrin tridecaacetate were carried out using the modifications suggested by Wagner[20] and Bax and Drobny.[21] Specifically, the phase cycling shown in Figure 1 is designed to remove axial peaks and contributions from NOE peaks and to suppress the P-type transitions; the transmitter can therefore be set in the center of the spectrum. Bax and Drobny[21] found a refocusing delay of 18 msec sufficient for a large range of coupling constants, but for the RCT experiment carried out on the α-cyclodextrin the refocusing delay τ was set to $(4J)^{-1}$. In addition, the mixing time τ was incremented in concert with the evolution period by adding a small fraction of the evolution time increment (typically $0.1 \times t_1$) to the delay τ for each experiment.[18,20] This had the effect of allowing a range of J values to be efficiently transferred. This technique was utilized in both the relay and double relay experiments using a starting value for both τs of 25 msec and ending with 34 msec. These τs correspond to J values between 8 and 12 Hz.

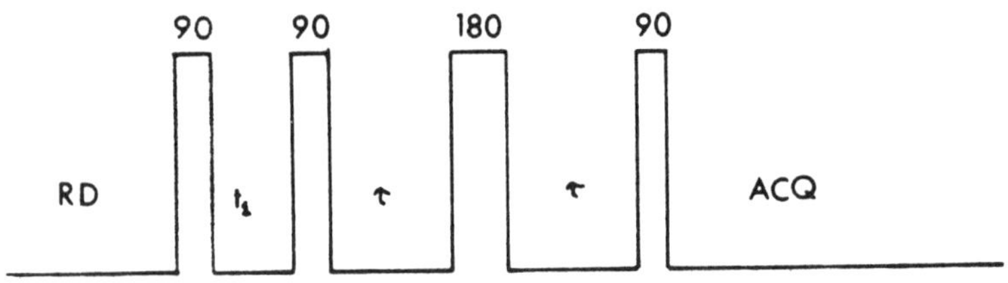

RCT
2D Relayed Coherence
Transfer Experiment

1 D5
2 P2/@A
3 D8
4 P2/@B
5 D3
6 P1/@B
7 D3
8 P2/@C
9 A@D
10 D2, Jump to 1
Phase
A = S
B = S + (S/8)
C = S + (2·(S/4)) + (S/8)
D = S + (2·(S/8))

Figure 1. Pulse sequence for two-dimensional homonuclear relayed coherence transfer (RCT) NMR experiment.

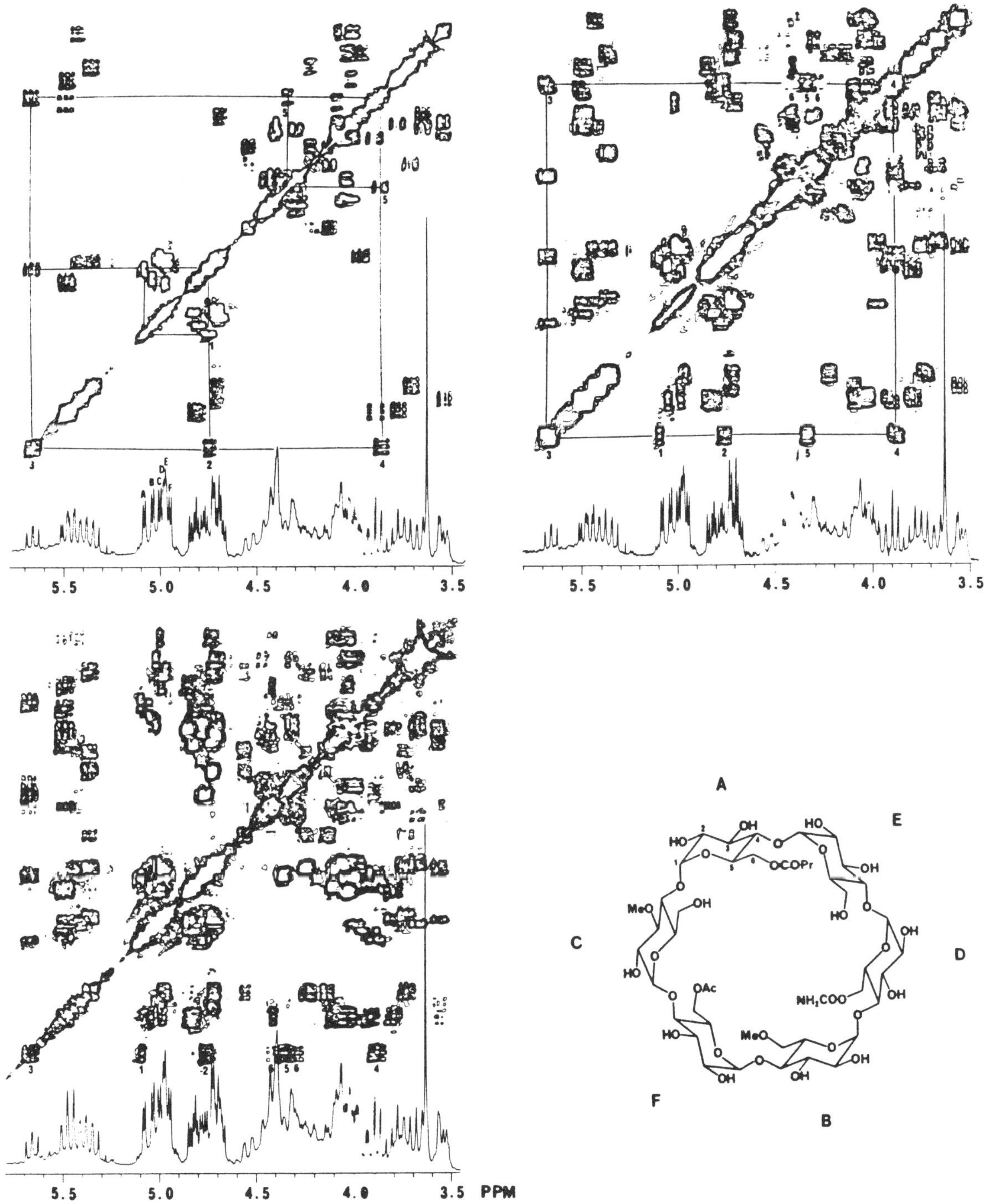

Figure 2. COSY16 (upper left), RCT (upper right), and RCT2 (lower right) spectra of a tridecaacetate derivative of a penta-O-substituted α-cyclodextrin from the cultured blue-green alga *Tolypothrix byssoidea*. The natural product is an O,O-dimethyl-α-cyclodextrin triester and its structure is shown at the lower right. Spectra were determined in chloroform-*d*.

The RCT and RCT2 spectra shown in Figure 2 were actually determined using Wagner's modified pulse sequence[20] as follows:

RCT

1 D5	10 D8
2 P2/@A	11 D3
3 DO 5, I LIMIT = 5	12 P2/@C
4 D8	13 A@D
5 D8	14 D2, Jump to 1
6 P2/@B	Phase
7 D8	A = S/4
8 D3	B = (2*(S/2))+S/4
9 P1/@B	C = (2*S)+(S/4)
	D = 1+(S/4)

P1 = 180 pulse; P2 = 90 pulse; D3 = refocusing delay time; D5 = post-acquisition delay time; D8 (initial delay time) = I8 (increment for D8 delays) = 1/10 DW (dwell time for acquisition)

For the RCT2 experiment, steps 7-12 were repeated using a different refocusing delay time (D4 = 20 msec instead of D3 = 25 msec). Data accumulation for RCT and RCT2 spectra takes longer than for a COSY spectrum for comparable signal-to-noise; the cross peaks for the relay spectra are always less intense. For the relay spectra in Figure 2, compared with the COSY, the number of scans per acquisition was doubled for the RCT experiment and quadrupled for the RCT2 experiment respectively.

SELECTIVE POLARIZATION TRANSFER SPECTROSCOPY

The most popular method for connecting proton spin-systems through quaternary carbons or heteroatoms is long-range shift correlation (HETCOR or CSCM) spectroscopy. Using this experiment the locations of the acetate, butyrate, and carbamate groups in the α-cyclodextrin tridecaacetate mentioned above were determined.[19] Compared with the normal ^1H-^{13}C CSCM spectrum, however, the long-range ^1H-^{13}C CSCM spectrum takes 50 times longer to determine. Since the intensities of the cross peaks in the long-range ^1H-^{13}C CSCM spectrum increase with longer spin-spin relaxation times, it is difficult to use this method on large molecules such as the α-cyclodextrin tridecaacetate, since the carbon T_2s are relatively short. On a 300-MHz instrument a meaningful long-range CSCM could not be obtained with a 50-mg sample, even after 2 days of data accumulation using optimum parameters; at 400 MHz, however, a long-range CSCM was determined after 24 hours of data accumulation. The corresponding one-bond CSCM was obtained with only 20 minutes of data accumulation at 400 MHz.

Selective polarization transfer spectroscopy or selective INEPT (SELINP)[17] is a much better method than long-range CSCM spectroscopy for macromolecules. Selective INEPT is a one-dimensional, T_2-independent experiment and is a natural extension of the standard refocused INEPT experiment.[22,23] Two modifications allow information to be transferred from protons to remote carbon nuclei. First, the non-selective proton pulses in the INEPT experiment are replaced by long ($90^{H-1} \geq 10$ msec, $\gamma H_2 = 25$ Hz) selective pulses centered on individual proton multiplets. Second, the two refocusing delays in the experiment are optimized for transfer between protons and carbons *via* long-range couplings rather than through one-bond couplings as in the usual INEPT experiment.

The pulse sequence shown in Figure 3 is basically the same as for the refocused INEPT experiment, but includes the aforementioned modification. The proton pulse widths are calibrated by either the off-resonance technique[24] or by the method suggested by Bax.[25]

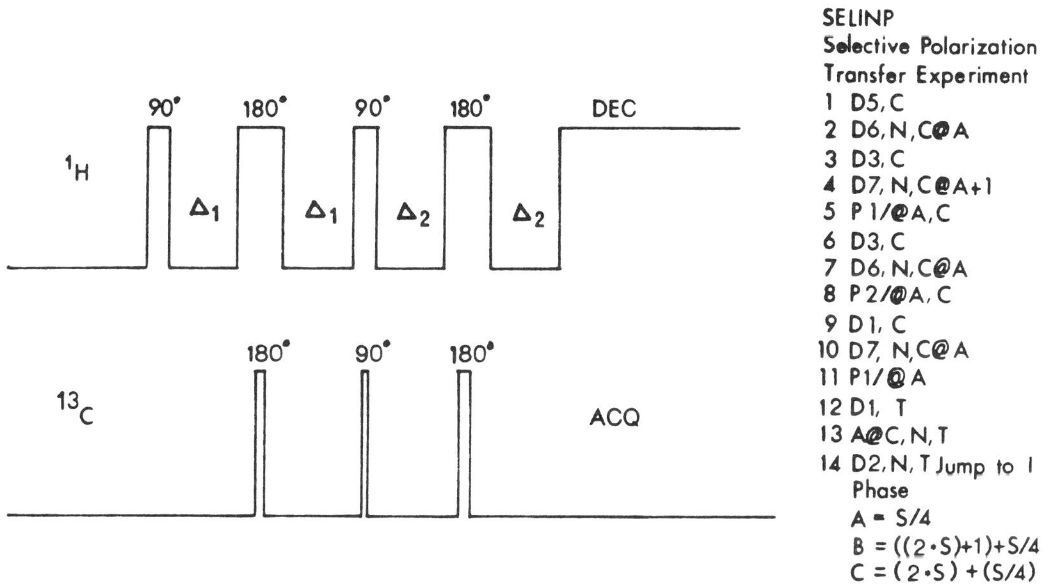

Figure 3. Pulse sequence for one-dimensional selective polarization transfer (selective INEPT) experiment.

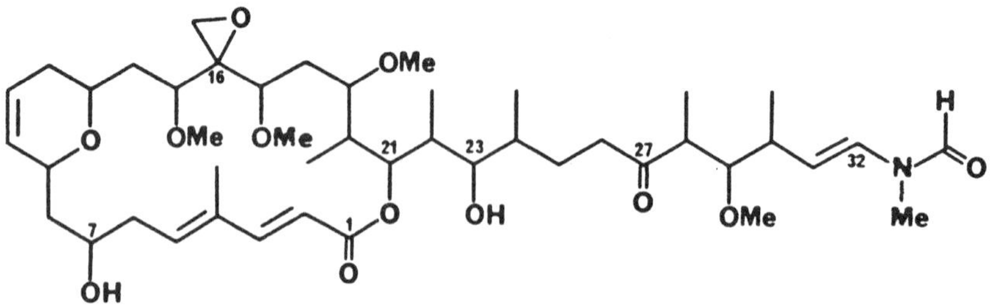

scytophycin B

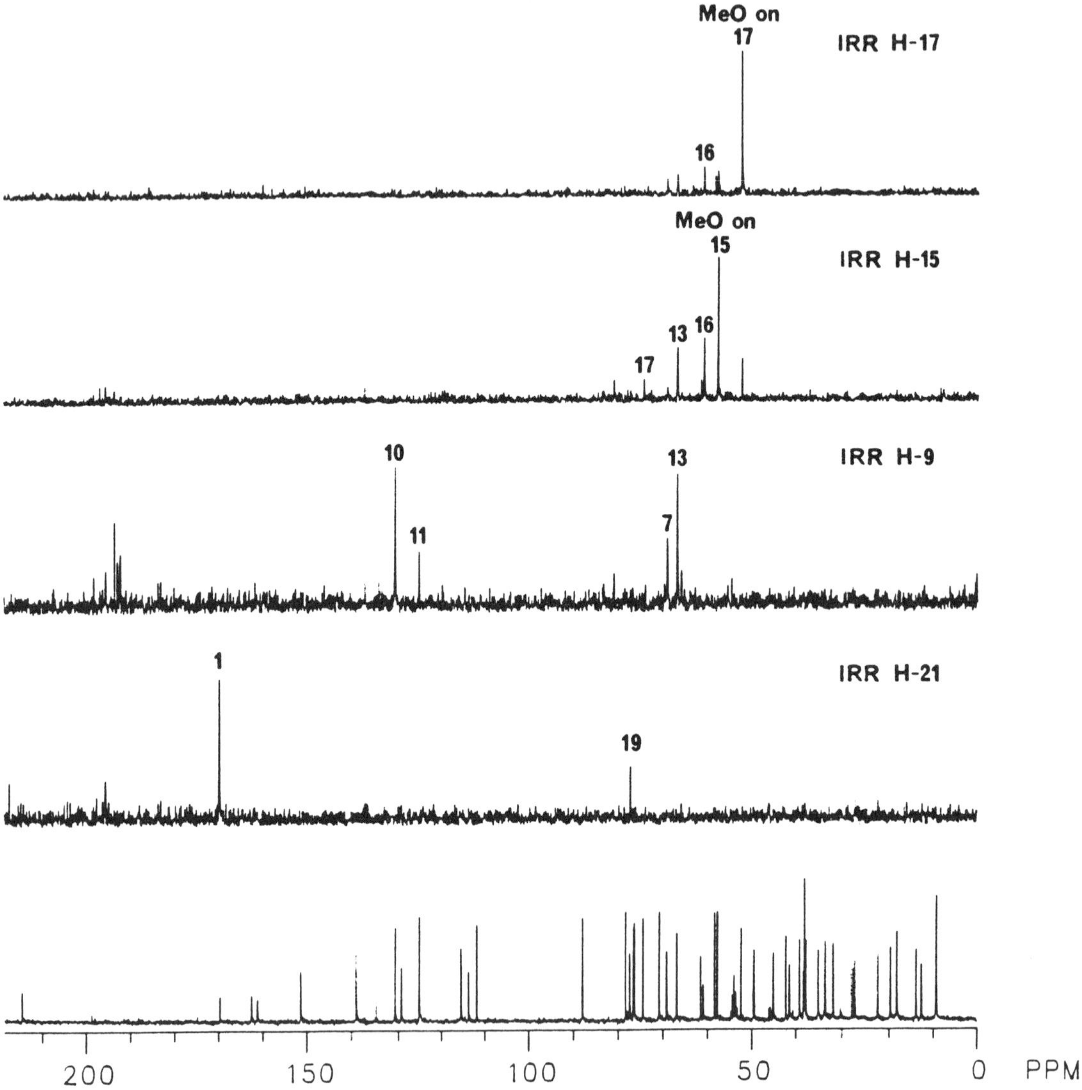

Figure 4. Proton-noise decoupled ^{13}C NMR spectrum (lower trace) and selective INEPT spectra (upper traces) of scytophycin B in dichloromethane-d_2.

In practice a sample of 1-^{13}C-acetic acid ($^{2}J_{H-C}$ = 6.7 Hz) will give accurate calibration of the soft proton pulse. For example, at a decoupler attenuator setting of 29 db on a Nicolet NT-300 spectrometer, the calibrated pulse width by either method yields a 90° proton pulse of 10.42 ± 0.2 msec. Exact proton frequencies are obtained by observing the ^{1}H spectrum through the decoupler coils of the ^{13}C probe. The refocusing delays used are essentially those suggested by Bax[17] (*i.e.*, Δ_1 = 25 msec and Δ_2 = 25 msec, 13 msec, and 10 msec for methine, equivalent methylene, or methyl groups, respectively).

Selective INEPT spectra for scytophycin B,[26] a potent cytotoxin and antifungal agent from the cultured blue-green alga *Scytonema pseudohofmanni*, are shown in Figure 4. The lower trace is the proton-noise decoupled ^{13}C-NMR spectrum of scytophycin B in dichloromethane-d_2 and the upper four traces represent the selective INEPT spectra obtained on irradiation of H-9, H-15, H-17, and H-21. When H-9 is irradiated, peaks are observed for C-7, C-10, C-11, and C-13. Visualization of the C-13 peak proves unambiguously that an ether oxygen connects C-9 and C-13. When H-15 is irradiated, signals are observed for C-13, the carbon of the methoxyl group on C-15, C-16, and C-17; however, no peak is observed for the methylene carbon on C-16. This spectrum, however, does establish connectivities of C-15 to the quaternary carbon of the epoxide ring (C-16) and C-17; it also shows unambiguously that a methoxyl group is attached to C-15. Similarly, irradiation of H-17 shows peaks for C-16 and the carbon of the methoxyl group on C-17. Finally when H-21 is irradiated, peaks are seen for C-1 and C-19. The C-1 peak proves rigorously that the ester oxygen connects C-1 and C-21.

Acknowledgments. High frequency NMR studies at the University of Hawaii have been supported by NSF Grants CHE83-03996 and CHE81-00240.

REFERENCES

1. Aue, W.P.; Bartholdi, E.; Ernst, R.R., *J. Chem. Phys.*, 1976, *64*, 2229.
2. Bax, A., "Two-Dimensional Nuclear Magnetic Resonance in Liquids", Delft University Press, Delft, Holland, 1982.
3. Morris, G.A., *Magn. Res. Chem.*, 1986, *24*, 371.
4. Turner, D.L., *Prog. Nucl. Magn. Res. Spectrosc.*, 1985, *17*, 281.
5. Kumar, A.; Hosur, R.V.; Chandrasekhar, K., *J. Magn. Reson.*, 1984, *60*, 1431
6. Bax, A.; Freeman, R., *J. Magn. Reson.*, 1981, *44*, 542.
7. Batta, G.; Liptak, A., *J. Am. Chem. Soc.*, 1984, *106*, 248.
8. Piantini, V.; Sorensen, V.W.; Ernst, R.R., *J. Am. Chem. Soc.*, 1982, *104*, 6800.
9. Rance, M.; Wagner, G.; Sorensen, O.W.; Wuthrich, K.; Ernst, R.R., *J. Magn. Reson.*, 1984, *59*, 250.
10. Bax, A.; Freeman, R., *J. Am. Chem. Soc.*, 1982, *104*, 1099.
11. Seto, H.; Furihata, K.; Otake, N.; Itoh, Y.; Takahashi, S.; Haneishi, T.; Ohuchi, M., *Tetrahedron Lett.*, 1984, *25*, 337.
12. Bothner-By, A.A.; Stephens, R.L.; Lee, J.-M.; Warren, C.D.; Jeanloz, R.W., *J. Am. Chem. Soc.*, 1984, *106*, 811.
13. Bax, A.; Davis, D.G., *J. Magn. Reson.*, 1985, *63*, 207.
14. Pachler, K.G.R.; Wessels, P.L., *J. Magn. Reson.*, 1973, *12*, 337.
15. Chalmers, A.A.; Pachler, K.G.R.; Wessels, P.L., *Org. Magn. Reson.*, 1974, *6*, 445.
16. Pachler, K.G.R.; Wessels, P.L., *J. Magn. Reson.*, 1977, *28*, 53.
17. Bax, A., *J. Magn. Reson.*, 1984, *57*, 314.
18. Eich, G.; Bodenhausen, G.; Ernst, R.R., *J. Am. Chem. Soc.*, 1982, *104*, 3732.
19. Entzeroth, M.; Moore, R.E.; Niemczura, W.P.; Patterson, G.M.L.; Shoolery, J., manuscript in preparation.
20. Wagner, G., *J. Magn. Reson.*, 1983, *55*, 151.
21. Bax, A.; Drobny, G., *J. Magn. Reson.*, 1985, *61*, 306.
22. Morris, G.A.; Freeman, R., *J. Am. Chem. Soc.*, 1979, *101*, 760.
23. Burum, D.P.; Ernst, R.R., *J. Magn. Reson.*, 1980, *39*, 163.

24. Thomas, D.M.; Bendall, M.R.; Pegg, D.T.; Doddrell, D.M.; Fields, J., *J. Magn. Reson.*, 1981, *42*, 298.
25. Bax, A., *J. Magn. Reson.*, 1983, *52*, 76.
26. Moore, R.E.; Patterson, G.M.L.; Mynderse, J.S.; Barchi, Jr, J.; Norton, T.R.; Furusawa, E.; Furusawa, S., *Pure Appl. Chem.*, 1985, *58*, 263.

Koji Nakanishi
Suntory Institute for Bio-organic Research, Wakayamadai, Shimamoto-cho, Mishima-gun, Osaka 618, Japan *and*
Department of Chemistry, Columbia University, New York, New York 10027, U.S.A.

New Isolation Methods and Spectroscopic Techniques

ISOLATION

As structure determinations become progressively more routine with dramatic advances in spectroscopic methods and X-ray crystallography, it has become feasible to handle compounds that were intractable a decade ago. These include biopolymers of various types, hormones, and other factors that are very unstable and/or exist in minute quantities but bear directly on the maintenance of life in nature. Similar revolutionary advances have changed isolation techniques centered around chromatography; the isolation process is unique, however, in that the availability of a bioactive factor in pure form is a critical first step in any scientifically sound analysis. Unless the factor to be studied is isolated without contamination, subsequent bioscientific results will usually be unreliable. It may even be that, unless purification is for some reason totally impossible, the labor and expense of biomedical, biological, biochemical, and other studies carried out on impure material will be wasted and lead to inconclusive discussions. As it becomes possible to deal with increasingly challenging isolation problems, the success or failure of a project depends frequently on whether or not the factor is obtained in pure form.

While synthetic or structural studies have general applications and provide intellectual satisfaction, such is not the case with isolation. The more challenging the isolation, the more likely it is to require years of frustrating trial and error, often based on empiricism or even instinct. The separation of two compounds may be achieved, for example, by adding a trace of a fourth solvent to a ternary HPLC solvent system. The isolation section of a lecture is usually of no particular interest to the audience and has no general appeal; nevertheless, it is crucial!

Probably the toughest isolation study we have carried out is that of the tunichromes,[1] the yellow, reducing blood pigments of the sea squirt or tunicate that sequesters vanadium from the ocean and concentrates it 10^6-10^7 fold.[2] Isolation studies of this pigment, noted even by Aristotle, began in 1911.[3] Numerous attempts were made, but the tunichromes resisted all efforts. The reason lies in the fact that although tunichromes are present in the blood of common marine animals, once the blood is collected from the heart, the tunichromes are extremely labile, particularly in the impure state, and brief exposure to air or a trace of humidity leads to browning (*i.e.*, polymerization, degradation, etc.). Consequently, all operations were carried out under dry oxygen-free argon using degassed solvents throughout.

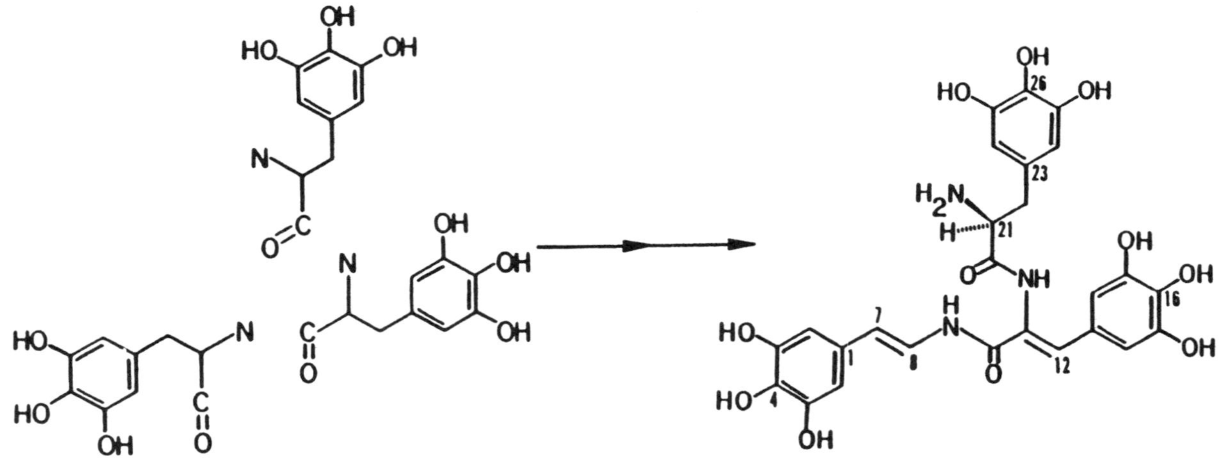

TUNICHROME B-1

1

Figure 1

During the 6-year period since we started these studies, approximately 6,000 tunicates were sacrificed, and it took fully 5 years to obtain 0.5 mg of pure tunichrome B-1 (TB-1).

As shown in Figure 1, the TB-1 structure can be formally derived from three molecules of hydroxy-DOPA. The overall isolation scheme is outlined in Figure 2. The blood was collected under argon and centrifuged, the centrifuged pellets were immersed in liquid nitrogen to lyse and freeze the cells and then were lyophilized for 3 days for complete dehydration; this procedure was followed in order to minimize water absorption. All fresh blood was processed to this stage without interruption. That is, the live tunicates were flown from Florida in lots of 1,000, brought in the evening from La Guardia Airport to the laboratory and processed immediately; collection of blood from 1,000 animals takes 5 hours when carried out by 10 people. The lyophilized pellets were ground in a mortar, suspended in the solvent shown, and applied to a 1-meter long LH-20 column. The LH-20 column was blown out when the tunichromes reached the end of the column, and the middle cut, consisting mostly of TB's, was extracted with methanol and precipitated by a series of solvent additions.

Analytical HPLC showed that the TB fraction consisted of at least three congeners (Figure 2). This was seen directly by a diode array detector that scans continuously from 190 nm to 370 nm every 0.2 sec as the HPLC is run; TB absorbs at 210 and 340 nm. It was very fortunate that we had a prototype apparatus for centrifugal counter-current chromatography (CCCC), since passing TB through HPLC results in 80% loss of material. The CCCC elution profile is shown in Figure 3, together with the very unusual solvent system. An advantage of this apparatus is that the elution mode can be reversed during operations so that fractions of various polarities can be efficiently eluted; the operation in Figure 3 took 9 hours.

The TB-1,2 fraction (5 mg) was finally passed through two semipreparative YMC gel ODS II columns (15 and 5 microns, both 25 x 250 mm) to give superb resolution and, for the first time, pure TB-1 (0.5 mg).

SECOND DERIVATIVE DIFFERENCE UV AND IR (SEDUV, SEDIR)[5]

As shown in Figure 4, second derivatization enhances resolution of spectral peaks; this is a well-known operation, carried out routinely by most modern spectrometers with computers. Strangely, the technique has rarely been used for structural studies. It was recently coupled successfully with computer subtraction to determine the structure of a mitomicyn C adduct obtained by reaction with an oligonucleotide at sub-milligram levels.[5]

The adduct structure is depicted in Figure 6; the other adduct is the 1β-isomer. I shall summarize the methodology in a series of figures.

Figure 5: The regular UV traces of alkylated guanine models are shown above and the SEDUV traces below. As shown in figure 5e, a single UV band at 215 nm is split into component peaks at 205 and 215 nm by SEDUV.

Figure 6: Difference SEDUV was used with microgram quantities of the adduct to determine the point of attachment of the mitosene moiety to guanine when this could not be done by NMR due to a lack of protons. The UV of adduct (A) was, therefore, taken and from it was subtracted the mitosene absorption (M). The residual UV (*i.e.*, A - M) was then compared to the reference set in Figure 5.

This figure clearly shows excellent agreement in the second derivative SEDUV with the N-7 adduct, particularly at short wavelengths; namely, peaks are at 205/216/245/285 for

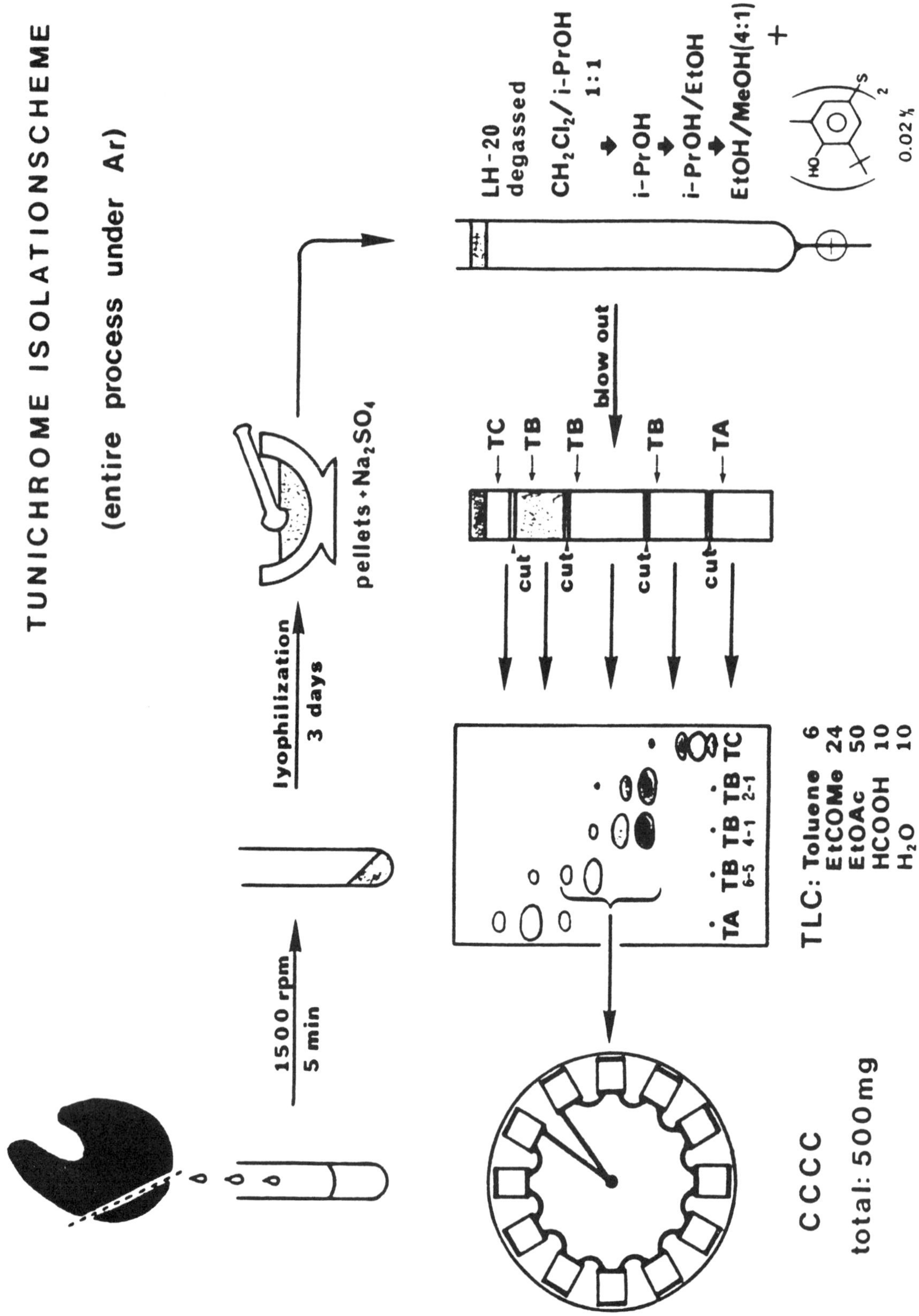
TUNICHROME ISOLATIONSCHEME
(entire process under Ar)
1500 rpm
5 min
lyophilization
3 days
pellets + Na_2SO_4
LH-20
degassed
CH_2Cl_2/i-PrOH
1:1
i-PrOH
i-PrOH/EtOH
EtOH/MeOH(4:1)
+
0.02 %
blow out
TC
TB
TB
TB
TA
cut
cut
cut
cut
TA
TB 6-5
TB 4-1
TB 2-1
TC
TLC: Toluene 6
EtCOMe 24
EtOAc 50
HCOOH 10
H_2O 10
CCCC
total: 500mg

Figure 2

CENTRIFUGAL COUNTERCURRENT CHROMATOGRAPHY

OF TUNICHROMES B .

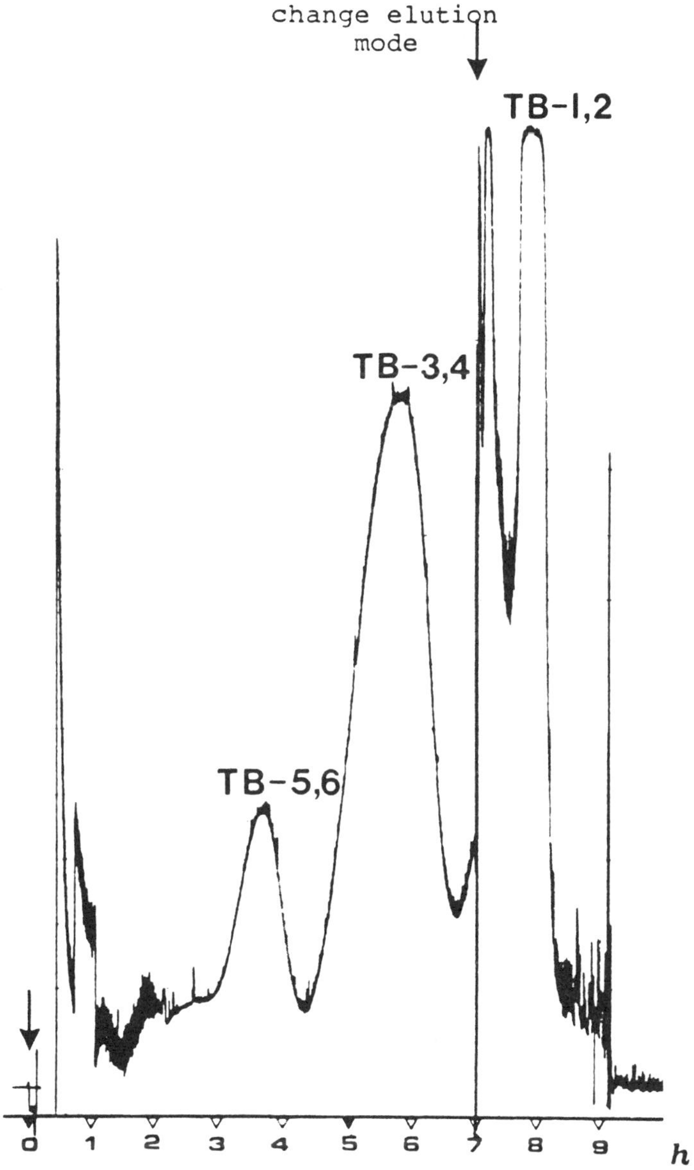

SOLVENT SYSTEM:

i-AMYLALCOHOL	8
n-BUTANOL	12
n-PROPANOL	10
WATER	30
FORMIC ACID	.25%
t-BUTYL SULFIDE	1%

ascending mode

2.4 ml/min

SPEED: 1000 rpm

BACK PRESSURE: 42 atm

UV 380 nm; 2.56 AUFS

----

1 cm/hr

Note: after elution of TB 3 the system was switched to descending mode.

Theoretical plates for

TB 3: N=750

TB 1: N=2000

Figure 3

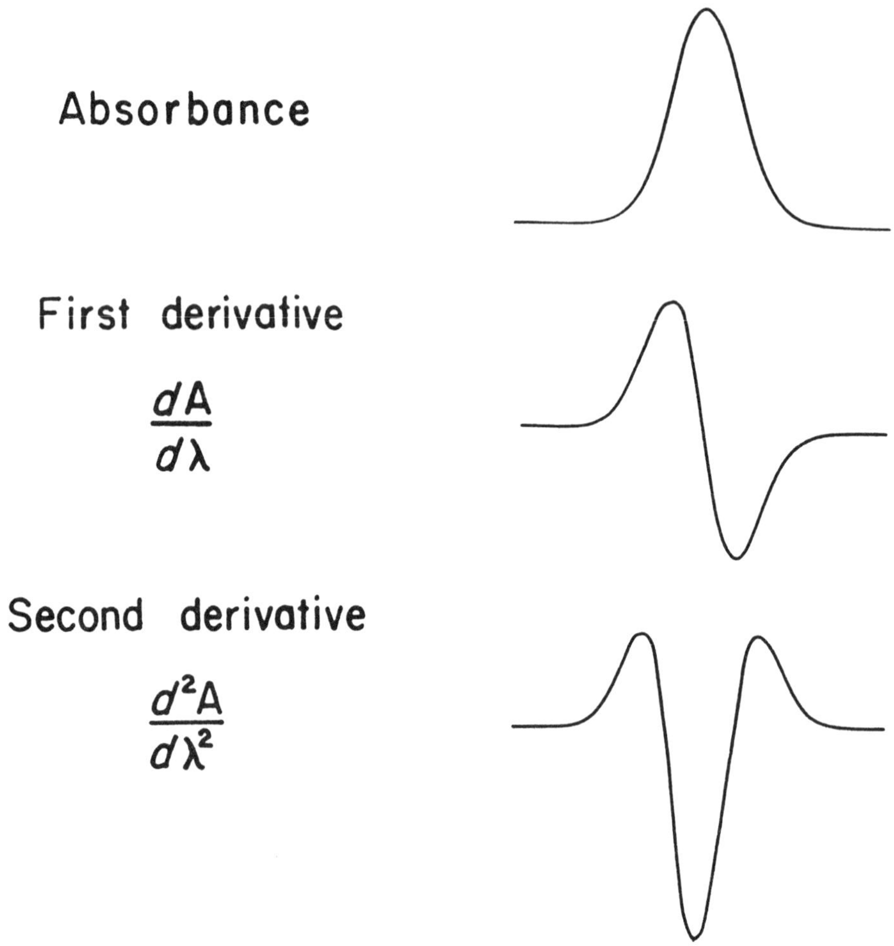
Absorbance
First derivative
$\frac{dA}{d\lambda}$
Second derivative
$\frac{d^2A}{d\lambda^2}$

Figure 4

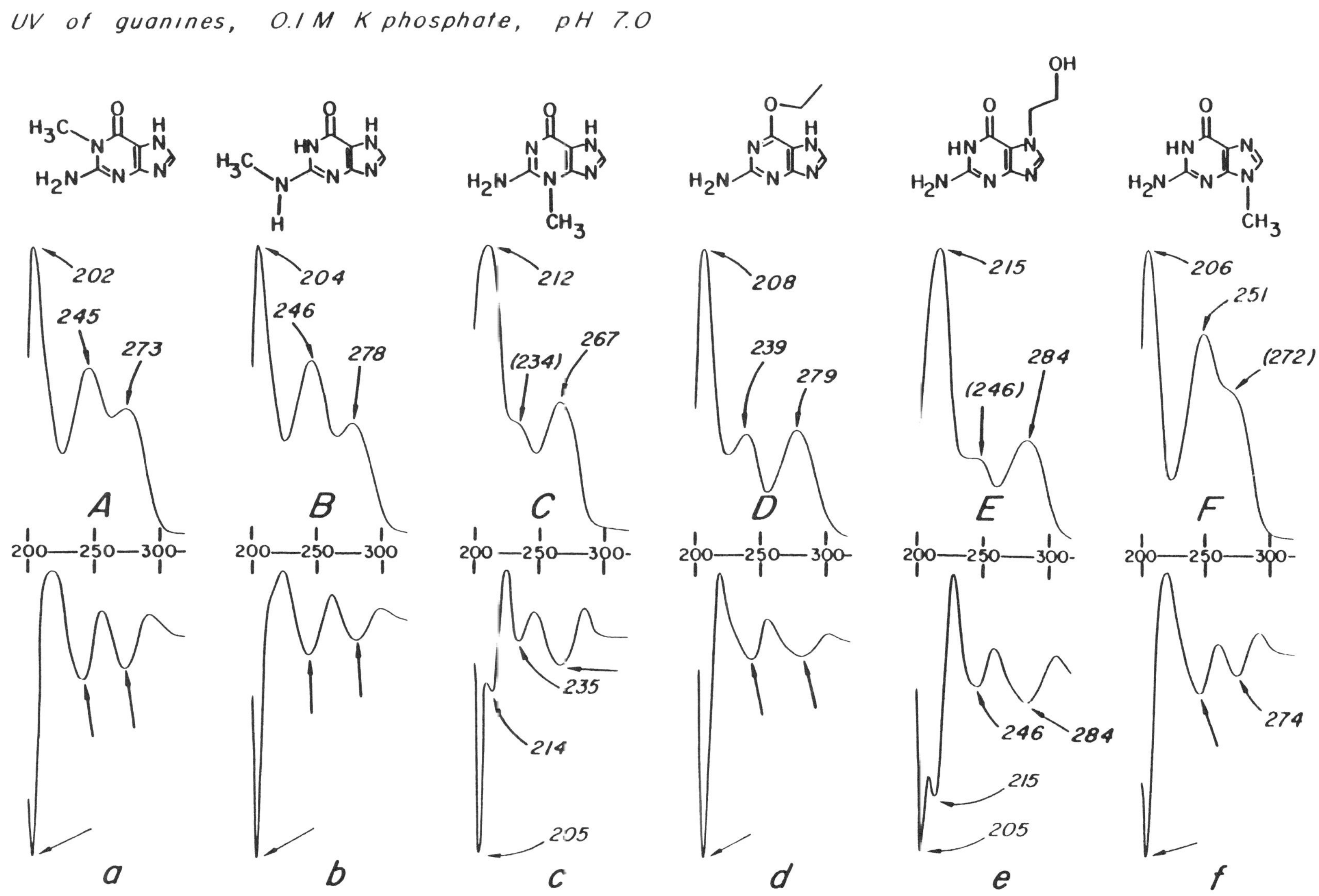
UV of guanines, 0.1 M K phosphate, pH 7.0
202
245
273
A
a
204
246
278
B
b
212
(234)
267
C
235
214
205
c
208
239
279
D
d
215
(246)
284
E
246
284
215
205
e
206
251
(272)
F
274
f
200—250—300

Figure 5

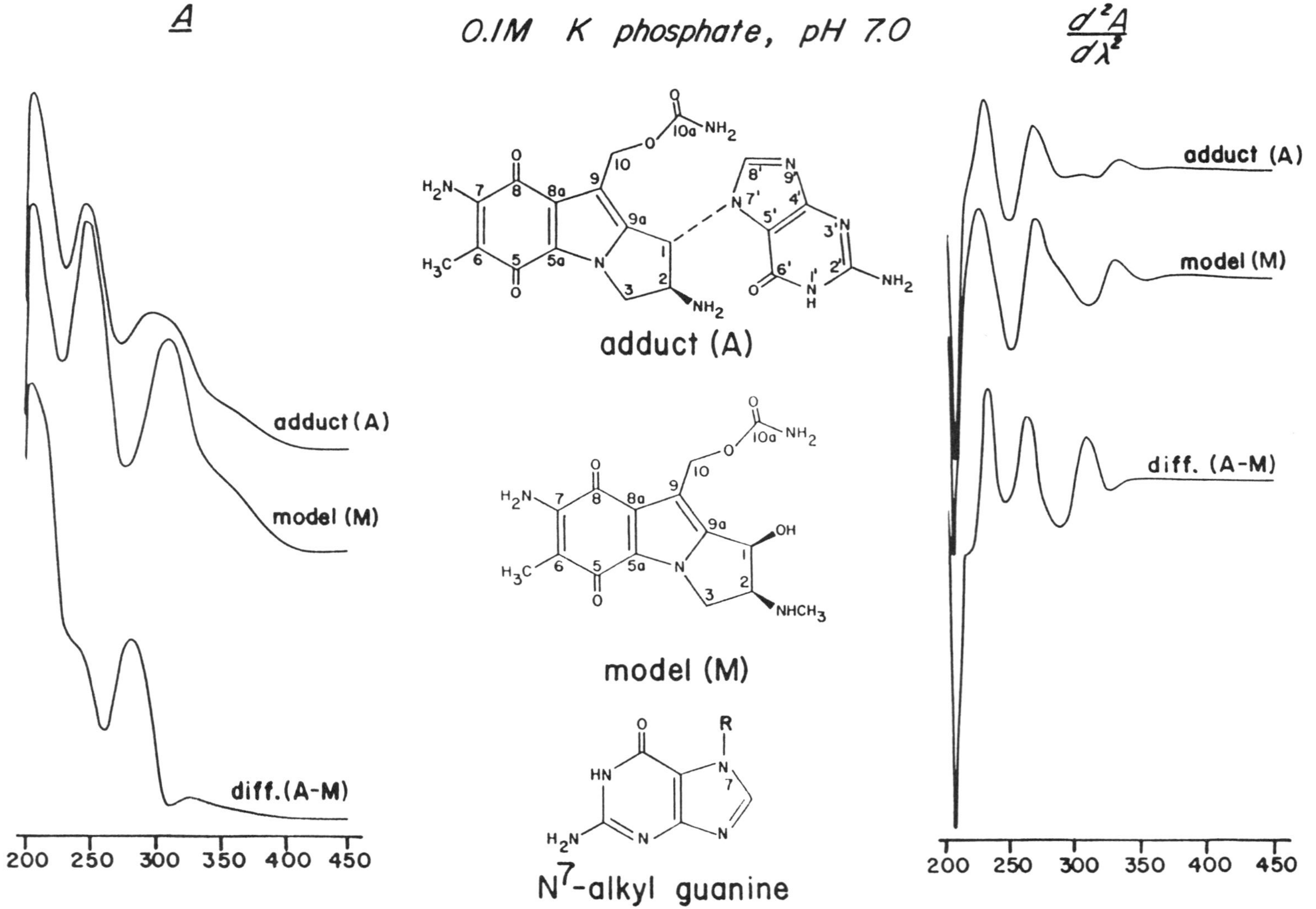
A
0.1M K phosphate, pH 7.0
d²A/dλ²
adduct (A)
model (M)
diff. (A-M)
200 250 300 350 400 450
N7-alkyl guanine

Figure 6

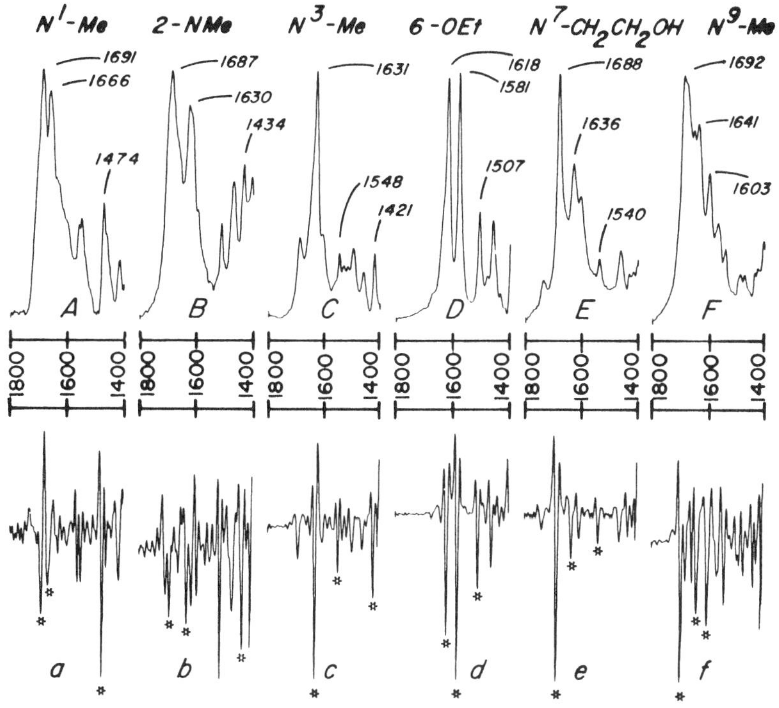

Figure 7

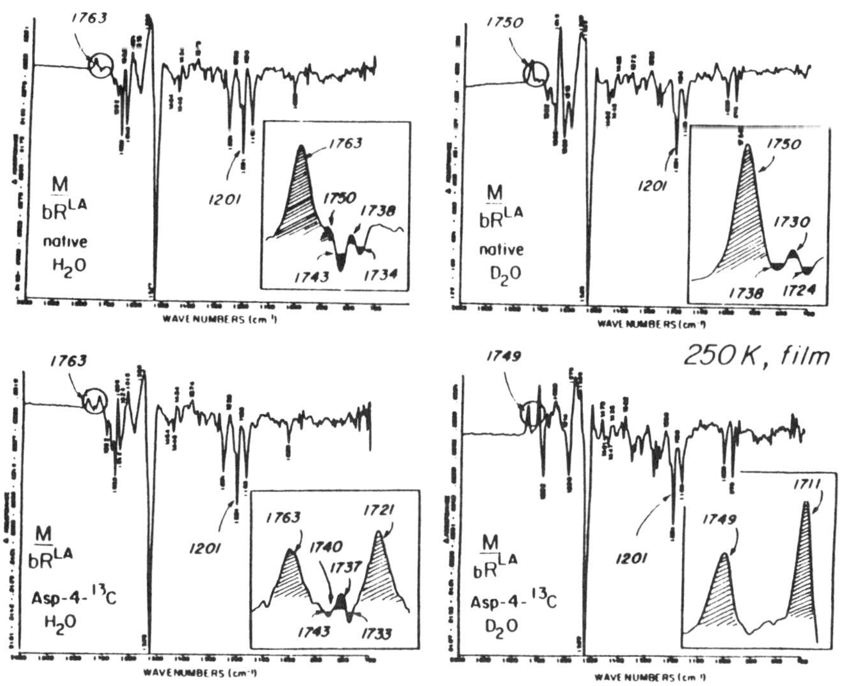

Figure 8

A-M and 205/215/246/284 for the reference in the difference SEDUV. Agreement in regular difference spectra is much less satisfactory.

Figure 7: FTIR spectra are shown for the standard set of alkylated guanines, as measured in CIRCLE attenuated total reflectance cells in DMSO-d_6 solution, in regular mode (above) and SEDIR mode (below). The SEDIR resolution is greatly enhanced. Here again when the difference spectra of adduct minus mitosene are compared in the two modes, there is far better agreement with Figure 7e (lower trace) than Figure 7E (upper trace).

Figure 8: Difference FTIR becomes an extremely powerful technique for measuring proteins and other biopolymers.[6] Figure 8 shows the difference spectrum between bacteriorhodopsin (bR, 26,000 daltons) and intermediate M, a crucial intermediate involved in proton pumping of bR (taken at 250K, hydrated film). The positive peak at 1763 cm^{-1} belonging to M (see upper left inset) shifts to 1750 in D_2O and hence represents either an Asp or Gln carboxyl. When difference FTIR of M/bR grown on medium containing 4-^{13}C-Asp is taken, the 1763 bond shifts to 1721 (lower left inset; the 1763 bond is due to residual regular Asp), which further shifts to 1711 in D_2O. The peak is thus Asp. This means that Asp is undergoing environmental change during the conversion of bR to M, and this should have a direct bearing on the clarification of the important mechanism of membrane proton translocation. The blacked out weaker absorptions, 1743/1734 for bR and 1738 for M (upper left inset) also shift to lower frequencies in D_2O but remain unchanged in the 4-^{13}C-Asp bR species; these peaks therefore represent Glu. This point is being checked currently with 5-^{13}C-Glu containing bR. This result indicates that some Glu residues are also undergoing environmental changes. The use of difference FTIR studies, complemented by resonance laser Raman measurements, indeed offers a most powerful approach for studying dynamic changes of biopolymers in solution.

REFERENCES

1. Bruening, R.C.; Oltz, E.M.; Furukawa, J.; Nakanishi, K.; Kustin, K., *J. Am. Chem. Soc.*, 1985, *107*, 5298.; *J. Nat. Prod.*, 1986, *49*, 193.
2. Kustin, K.; Ladd, K.V.; McLeod, G.C., *J. Gen. Physiol.*, 1975, *65*, 315.
3. Henze, M., *Hoppe-Seyler's Z. Physiol. Chem.*, 1911, *72*, 494.
4. Murayama, W.; Kobayashi, T.; Kosuge, Y.; Yano, H.; Nunogaki, Y.; Nunogaki, K., *J. Chrom.*, 1982, *239*, 643; Bruening, R.C.; Derguini, F.; Okuda, R.; Nakanishi, K., Abstr. Pap. - Annu. Chem. Soc. 189th ANYL 165 (1985). The CCCC apparatus is now commercially manufactured by Sanki Engineering Ltd., 2-6-10 Imazato, Nagaokakyo, Kyoto, Japan.
5. Verdin, G.; Nakanishi, K., *J. Am. Chem. Soc.*, 1985, *107*, 6118, 6120.
6. Bagley, K.; Dollinger, G.; Eisenstein, L.; Singh, A.K.; Zimanyi, L., *Proc. Natl. Acad. Sci., USA*, 1979, *79*, 4972.
7. Derguini, F.; Dunn, D.; Eisenstein, L.; Nakanishi, K.; Odashima, K.; Rao, V.J.; Sastry, L.; Termini, J., *Pure Appl. Chem.*, 1985, *58*, 719.

Arnold Brossi, Bernhard Schönenberger
Medicinal Chemistry Section, Laboratory of Chemistry, National Institute of Arthritis, Diabetes, and Digestive and Kidney Diseases, National Institutes of Health, Bethesda, Maryland 20892, U.S.A.

Enantiospecificity and Biological Activity of Natural Products

Most chiral natural products are optically pure isomers. Comparison studies with the unnatural enantiomers reveal, in most cases, significant differences in the biological activity of the two. Optically active natural products, therefore, should be viewed in the same way as natural amino acids or carbohydrates.

The point may be illustrated by several examples. The alkaloid morphine, which as natural (-)-morphine binds to opiate receptors, has profound effects on the CNS, resulting in analgesia, addiction, and physical dependence,[1] whereas the unnatural (+)-morphine obtained from sinomenine[2] or by total synthesis[3] does not show such properties.[2,4] The antibiotic griseofulvin when tested as the unnatural (-)-enantiomer[5] did not exhibit the potent antifungal activity of the natural (+)-enantiomer,[5] and (+)-emetine prepared by total synthesis is much inferior as an antiprotozoal agent to natural (-)-emetine.[6] Different biological properties were also reported for R-(-)-apomorphine, showing agonist activity in assays measuring binding to D-2-dopamine receptors, and S-(+)-apomorphine, which behaved as an antagonist in this assay.[7] Binding to chiral receptor molecules and enzyme-controlled metabolic conversion of chiral compounds *in vivo* are probable reasons for these differences. It is prudent to suggest, therefore, that total synthesis of a biologically active chiral molecule should be directed from the beginning to a synthesis of its enantiomers, allowing an assessment of the enantiospecific nature of biological action. Testing of racemates without comparison to one enantiomer as a standard does not seem logical and will add biased data to a literature already loaded with such data.

The synthesis of unnatural (+)-physostigmine, accomplished by Kobayashi and by Robinson *et al.*, included a low-yield optical resolution step;[8] practical preparation required a better approach. The formation of urea diastereomers by chiral benzyl isocyanates is frequently used to determine the optical purity of amines, where the ratio of diastereomers is measured by ^{1}H NMR or HPLC.[9] This procedure has become a preparative method for resolving chiral secondary amines. The urea diastereomers are separated on a multi-gram scale by column chromatography, HPLC, or by crystallization, then degraded in refluxing alcohols in the presence of one or more equivalents of the sodium alcoholate to give the desired optically pure amines and neutral by-products, originating from the chiral benzylamine.[10] In several cases, the yield of the individual enantiomers after fragmentation exceeded 40%, and their optical purity was assessed to be greater than 97% by HPLC. The reaction sequence, carried out with (±)-*N*1-

noreseroline-*O*-methyl ether obtained by total synthesis, readily afforded the desired optically active enantiomers in high yield and excellent optical purity.[11]

Another example of this novel resolution is the case of (±)-salsolidine,[12] a simple isoquinoline alkaloid that occurs in nature as a racemate as well as in the form of both optical antipodes.[13] After one crystallization from dichloromethane-diisopropyl ether, the urea diastereomers obtained by reaction of (±)-salsolidine and R-(+)-α-methyl benzyl isocyanate in chloroform afforded one of the diastereomers in 46% yield and essentially optically pure (HPLC, 98%). The mother liquor, therefore, was enriched in the other diastereomer (HPLC, 92%). Both diastereomers decomposed in refluxing 2 M sodium 1-butanoxide in butanol; the usual work-up yielded (-)- and (+)-salsolidine of established absolute configurations.[14] Recrystallization of the hydrochloride salts prepared from the two alkaloids allowed further optical purification and gave data identical to those reported.[14] It is hoped that organic chemists studying bioactive natural products will have ample opportunities to apply this new method to the resolution of secondary amines.

REFERENCES

1. Jacquet, Y.F.; Klee, W.A.; Rice, K.C.; Iijima, I.; Minamikawa, J., *Science (Washington, D.C.)*, 1977, *198*, 842.
2. Goto, K., "Sinomenine, an Optical Antipode of Morphine Alkaloids", Kitasato Institute, Tokyo, 1964, pp 1-142.
3. Rice, K.C., in "The Chemistry and Biology of Isoquinoline Alkaloids", J.D. Phillipson, M.F. Roberts, M.H. Zenk, Eds., Springer Verlag, Berlin, 1985, pp 191-203.
4. (+)-Morphine prepared by the Rice total synthesis is presently being studied pharmacologically at various institutions.
5. Brossi, A.; Baumann, M.; Burkhardt, F., *Helv. Chim. Acta*, 1962, *45*, 1292.
6. Brossi, A.; Brener, Z.; Pellegrino, J.; Stohler, H.; Frey, J.R., *Experientia*, 1960, *16*, 64.
7. Neumeyer, J.L., in Ref. 3, pp 146-170.
8. (a) Kobayashi, T., *Justus Liebigs Ann. Chem.*, 1938, *536*, 143.
   (b) Dale, F.J.; Robinson, B., *J. Pharm. Pharmacol.*, 1970, *22*, 889.
9. Rice, K.C.; Brossi, A., *J. Org. Chem.*, 1980, *45*, 592.
10. Experimental details on this resolution will be given in a full paper which is in preparation.
11. Brossi, A., *J. Nat. Prod.*, 1985, *48*, 878.
12. Prepared by standard reduction of 1,2-dehydrosalsolidine with sodiumborohydride in methanol. See *Org. Synt.*, 1977, *56*, 3.
13. Kametani, T., "The Chemistry of the Isoquinoline Alkaloids", Elsevier, Amsterdam, 1969, pp 25-25.
14. Battersby, A.R.; Edwards, T.P., *J. Chem. Soc.*, 1960, 1214.

Section V

Financial Support for Research on Bio-Active and Pharmaceutical Products from the Sea

Wiliam F. Raub, Melvin S. Fish
Office of Extramural Research and Training, Office of the Director, National Institutes of Health,
Bethesda, Maryland 20892, U.S.A.

Funding of Drug Development and Research on Marine Natural Products by the N.I.H.

INTRODUCTION

Pharmacologically active substances derived from marine organisms are relevant to the missions of several of the National Institutes of Health (NIH). Although there is no NIH program focused exclusively on the discovery and study of such substances, the agency fosters a substantial body of research and development in this area. This paper presents brief background information on the NIH, highlights its interests in drug development in general and marine natural products in particular, and summarizes some of the scientific and administrative considerations that are expected to guide its future efforts.

THE NATIONAL INSTITUTES OF HEALTH (NIH)

The NIH exists to improve human health by conducting research in its laboratories and clinics and by funding research in universities and colleges, non-profit research institutes, other government laboratories, hospitals, and small and large businesses. The NIH mission spans almost all forms of human disease and disability, and the various components of the agency approach their respective legal mandates not only by fostering studies targeted toward improved prevention, diagnosis, treatment, and rehabilitation, but also by promoting basic research on life processes. The array of NIH-funded projects ranges from theoretical studies through laboratory and clinical investigations to field trials and surveys.

DRUG DEVELOPMENT

Essentially every NIH component that conducts or funds research is involved in some aspect of drug development. The National Cancer Institute is perhaps the most comprehensive in its operations; its quest for new chemotherapeutic and chemopreventive agents spans the spectrum from broadly directed screening via *in vitro* tests to large-scale clinical trials. Three other Institutes routinely pursue selected leads all the way through clinical trials; these are the National Institute of Allergy and Infectious Diseases (vaccines and antiviral drugs), the National Institute of Child Health and Human Development (contraceptives), and the National Institute of Neurological and Communicative Disorders and Stroke (antiepileptic drugs). All the NIH components regularly conduct or fund research projects on biologically active natural substances:

namely, the isolation, identification, characterization, laboratory synthesis, use as pharmacological probes, elucidation of biosynthetic pathways, elucidation of the mechanism of action, and assessment of pharmacologic and toxicologic properties as manifested in laboratory animals and human subjects.

NATURAL PRODUCTS OF MARINE ORIGIN

A. General. Because NIH activities related to drug development are spread throughout the fabric of its programs and because research on marine natural products generally is neither managed nor classified separately, there is no practical way to make a precise and complete tabulation of ongoing projects. However, a conservative analysis by the NIH Division of Research Grants reveals 104 research projects on marine natural products with an aggregate expenditure of over $10 million. A similarly conservative analysis reveals an additional 133 research projects (at a cost of approximately $14 million) focused on natural products of non-marine origin and an additional 115 projects (at a cost of over $12 million) involving the chemical synthesis of natural products from various sources. Most of these projects are funded by research grants to scientists in institutions of higher education, but some work in each of these areas is being carried out in NIH laboratories. Virtually all of the studies are the result of independent initiatives by individual investigators.

B. Specific Examples. (1) National Cancer Institute (NCI). Marine natural products traditionally have been included among the substances tested by the NCI for antitumor or cytotoxic activity. The NCI reports that to date it has received over 15,000 extracts from marine organisms and currently has one substance of marine origin in clinical trials (didemnin B). A description of the NCI program in drug development has been presented by Driscoll (Cancer Treatment Reports 68:63-76, 1984) and by Marsoni and Wittes (Cancer Treatment Reports 68:77-85, 1984).

Among the ongoing research grants funded by the NCI, three seem noteworthy: (a) studies of antitumor agents extracted from blue-green algae (R.E. Moore, University of Hawaii, CA12623); (b) studies of the antineoplastic properties of novel cyclic peptides extracted from marine tunicates (C.M. Ireland, University of Utah; CA36622); and (c) clinical testing of ω-3 fatty acids from fish oils as chemopreventive agents for breast cancer (M.P. Osbourne, Memorial Hospital for Cancer and Allied Diseases, New York; CA38401). Moreover, the first of these projects was cited recently by an NCI advisory group as part of the basis for its recommendation that the NCI do more to facilitate studies of algal extracts. The group called for an initiative to collect, isolate, and culture blue-green algae and to provide extracts for antitumor or cytotoxicity screening by the NCI. The advisory group also called for two related initiatives: a project to isolate, ferment, and prepare testable extracts from marine microorganisms and a project to collect and classify samples of a wide variety of marine organisms preparatory to extractions and testing of substances having possible chemotherapeutic potential. Solicitation of contract proposals recently occurred in all three areas.

(2) National Heart, Lung and Blood Institute (NHLBI) and National Institute of Arthritis, Diabetes, and Digestive and Kidney Diseases (NIADDK). The NHLBI and the NIADDK have a common interest with the NCI in the effects of marine lipids contained in human diets. For example, NHLBI funds studies of the effects of dietary fish oils on elevated blood lipids (W.E. Connor, Oregon Health Sciences University; HL25687; and B.C. Bullock, Wake Forest University; HL30342). Another NHLBI-funded project explores the effects of dietary fish oils on autoimmune phenomena related to atherosclerosis and glomerulonephritis (N.J. Alexander, Oregon Regional Primate Research Center; HL31517). An NIADDK-funded project focuses on the roles of prostaglandins and leukotrienes in inflammatory rheumatic diseases, especially with

respect to how inflammation and immune responses are affected by marine lipids in the diet (D.R. Robinson, Massachusetts General Hospital; AM19427).

(3) National Institute of Allergy and Infectious Diseases (NIAID). The NIAID, as its name suggests, is the focal point within the NIH for research related to antimicrobial and antiviral agents. Two projects illustrate this activity well: (a) studies of antimicrobial and antiviral compounds derived from marine tunicates and sponges (K.L. Rinehart, Jr., University of Illinois; AIO4769) and (b) studies of antibiotics derived from marine algae and bacteria (D.J. Faulkner, U.C.-San Diego; AI11969).

(4) National Institute of Dental Research (NIDR). The NIDR shares with the NIAID a mission interest in antimicrobial and antiviral agents. An example of this is the NIDR-funded project entitled "Marine Microalgae with Antiherpes Properties" (R.J. Lewis, Neushul Mariculture, Inc., Goleta, CA; DE06899). This project is funded under the NIH Small Business Innovation Research Program (see "Prospects" below).

The NIDR shares with the National Eye Institute (NEI) an interest in the adhesive properties of a protein from the mussel *Mytilus edulis*. NEI funds a study to assess the efficacy of this bioadhesive in the transplantation of corneal endothelial cells (P. Picciano, Biopolymers, Inc., Farmington, CT; EY05713). NIDR funds a more wide-ranging study under the NIH Small Business Innovation Research Program (C.V. Benedict, Biopolymers, Inc., Farmington, CT; DE07266).

(5) National Institute of General Medical Sciences (NIGMS). The NIGMS funds a substantial fraction of NIH grants for basic and targeted research in pharmacology. Among these many projects, four place particular emphasis on marine natural products: (a) studies of the biosynthesis of unusual sterols from lower marine animals (C. Djerassi, Stanford University; GM06840); (b) studies of biosynthesis of saxitoxin, gonyautoxins, tetrodotoxin, and related substances in marine organisms (Y. Shimizu, University of Rhode Island; GM24425); (c) studies of the biological and chemical properties of the toxins Latrunculin A and B derived from Red Sea sponges (I. Spector, SUNY, Stony Brook; GM32776); and (d) determinations of the primary structure of neurotoxins from sea anemones and their detailed interaction with sodium channels (W.R. Kem, University of Florida; GM32848).

The Institute and the NIH Division of Research Resources also facilitate drug development from natural products by funding much of the research, development, and equipment acquisition associated with the determination of molecular structure (*e.g.* mass spectrometry, nuclear magnetic resonance, X-ray crystallography, and computer graphics).

(6) National Institute of Neurological and Communicative Disorders and Stroke (NINCDS). NINCDS-funded research involving marine natural products complements the NIGMS interest in molecular interactions. Three projects illustrate this: (a) studies of the structure and action of polypeptide axonal toxins from the marine worm *Cerebratulus lacteus* (K.M. Blumenthal, University of Cincinnati; NS14368); (b) studies of the effects of tetrosotoxin on muscle and nerve receptors (C.-Y. Kao, SUNY Downstate Medical Center; NS14551); and (c) use of the purified acetylcholine receptor from Torpedo electric tissue to study the molecular mechanism of toxin effects (J. Schmidt, SUNY, Stony Brook; NS18839).

PROSPECTS

It seems highly likely that the NIH's role in developing drugs from marine natural products will grow in the years immediately ahead. Given the burgeoning interest in this area within the scientific community, more individual investigators can be expected to submit grant applications. Given the many scientists skilled in natural products chemistry and the ever-increasing power of chemical technology, a substantial number of these applications can be expected to succeed. Moreover, the challenge to find a cure for Acquired Immune Deficiency Syndrome, provides additional motivation to seek pharmacologically effective substances from the sea .

Research on marine natural products and the pursuit of their commercial possibilities should be facilitated by the new collaboration among Government, universities, non-profit research institutes, and industry. Since 1981, businesses have been eligible to receive research grants from the NIH under terms essentially identical to those that apply to non-profit organizations. In particular, all domestic awardees now retain first rights to inventions they produce with funds from agencies of the U.S. Government. Also, since 1983, the NIH and other agencies have operated a Small Business Innovation Research Program (Public Law 97-219) under which funds are set aside to ensure that meritorious research and development projects proposed by companies are funded with a view to creating new commercial products and services. Throughout the last decade, particularly in the wake of the emergence of genetic engineering, an array of productive relationships has grown up involving universities and other non-profit organizations on the one hand and commercial organizations, both large and small, on the other.

The prospects for successfully tapping the latent pharmacological potential of marine organisms seem bright. The NIH is well-positioned to continue its catalytic role and is eager to do so.

David H. Attaway
United States Department of Commerce, National Oceanographic and Atmospheric Administration, National Sea Grant College Program, 6010 Executive Boulevard, Rockville, Maryland 20852, U.S.A.

Biotechnology in the National Sea Grant College Program

The National Sea Grant College Program sponsors a small but highly productive research effort in marine pharmacology as part of a larger marine biotechnology program. About $2,000,000 in federal funds and $1,000,000 in matching funds are invested annually in marine biotechnology. I will sketch the bounds of this program, describe some of its recent advances, and suggest some opportunities for fundamental research that will aid the long-term development of marine resources.

Biotechnology is the application of scientific and engineering principles to the processing of materials produced by biological agents in order to provide goods and services.[1] Exclusive of traditional agriculture, applications of biotechnology in water treatment and purification (primarily of domestic sewage) now account for the largest volume of material processed. The production of beer and spirits, cheese and other dairy products, baker's yeast, organic acids, and antibiotics follow in order of decreasing volume and value. These applications of biotechnology are based on the use of microorganisms and are of great importance to the economy and to society's well-being. In the United States, for example, the market value of antibiotics and other fine chemicals produced biotechnologically is approximately $8 billion annually.[2]

Biotechnology is not new, but with new techniques for designing genetic change and for cloning cell lines, it has become of increased interest to both scientists and businessmen. The ability to change the genetic complement of organisms without the slow process of selective breeding offers almost unlimited possibilities for harnessing the biochemical processes of living systems for medical, agricultural, and commercial purposes. Commonly occurring bacteria already have been redesigned for the production, through mass culture, of interferon, hormones, vaccines, diagnostic reagents, and other medically useful substances.

Applications of biotechnology to the use and development of marine resources have only recently been widely recognized. The scientific basis for application of modern genetics, physiology, biochemistry, and engineering to the commercial use of marine organisms is sketchy. Opportunities for fundamental and applied marine research relevant to the development of marine biotechnology span several disciplines and areas of research. Harnessing the genetics and biochemistry of living marine organisms will require the development of new technology, including engineering and biochemical engineering, as well as careful consideration of economic and social issues. Yet the basic research for this new technology is relatively inexpensive, and a significant portion of it logically belongs in academic institutions.

In speaking of future sources of organic raw materials, I.S. Shapiro, Chairman of E.I. duPont de Nemours & Company, suggested a broad role for academic institutions.[3] "They could work across the disciplinary boundaries, look at the interlocking economic and political factors as well as the technical data coming from scientists and engineers, and try to set forth in a rational way the options that exist and the consequences of each." Mr. Shapiro points further to the need for responsible government leadership toward a strong future economic base, rather than toward short-term expedients. "Thus we must work together across the boundaries of nations and institutions, through research, through development, and through education, to be responsible stewards of the raw materials at hand, and to create new resources for the future." R.W. Schmitt, Senior Vice President for Corporate Research and Development of the General Electric Company, pointed out that, "The most important role for government in creating conditions for commercial innovation is to support universities in their efforts to generate research and provide manpower."[4] He suggests that the government should stress the growth of sunrise science and technology or fast-moving areas of research. Some of the opportunities for such sunrise science relating to marine resources can be considered in the following categories: biochemistry and pharmacology, genetic engineering, biochemical engineering, microbiology and phycology.

BIOCHEMISTRY AND PHARMACOLOGY

Terrestrial plants and microorganisms are the direct or indirect sources of most pharmaceuticals whether synthetically or biotechnologically produced. Almost all of the antibiotics in current use are secondary metabolites of microorganisms and are invaluable in medicine. Marine organisms, especially microorganisms, have been little explored for useful organic substances. However, results so far show the sea to be a rich source of secondary metabolites with unique combinations of elements, as well as physical, chemical, and biological properties not encountered in terrestrial materials.

Primary metabolites such as unsaturated fatty acids, which are components of fish oils and microalgae, may be of tremendous importance in human health. For example, evidence is accumulating that eicosapentaenoic acid may help ward off inflammatory and cardiovascular diseases. Other primary metabolites of marine organisms, such as the polymers carageenan, alginic acid, and agar agar, already are used widely in the pharmaceutical and food industries; they are produced annually in hundred-million-dollar quantities. Yet, little organized and fundamental study has focused on polymers of marine organisms, particularly microorganisms.

The high incidence of biological activity associated with secondary metabolites of marine organisms indicates the potential richness of the marine environment as a source of useful compounds for medicine and agriculture, in the latter case as pesticides or regulators of plant growth. The emphasis in research to date has been on determining the chemical structures of the varied compounds discovered by the marine natural products chemists in the easily collected members of coastal fauna and flora. Chemists have assigned scores of novel and exotic structures such as that of okadaic acid, a C_{38} polyether fatty acid first isolated from sponges,[5] which was characterized by X-ray diffraction studies and later shown to be produced by the dinoflagellate *Prorocentrum lima*.[6] It is a potentially useful compound that inhibits the growth of KB cells derived from a human tumor.

In general, the biological functions and pharmacological or medicinal properties of these extraordinary substances have not been thoroughly investigated. The modest but sophisticated efforts in this direction in the National Sea Grant College Program, mainly those of Dr. R. Jacobs of the University of California at Santa Barbara, have produced promising leads and defined new mechanisms of pharmacological action. Some discoveries are in the early stages of commercialization. Manoalide, for example, isolated from a Pacific sponge,[7] exhibits a number of properties of pharmacological interest[8] and could be a model for a new class of nonsteroidal, anti-inflammatory drugs.

Stypoldione, a marine cytotoxin extracted from seaweed, was discovered during investigations by a research team headed by Dr. W. Fenical at the Scripps Institute of Oceanography.[9] Cytotoxins, as their name suggests, are compounds that kill cells; the drug vincristine, for example, a natural drug derived from a terrestrial plant, is a cytotoxin used in cancer chemotherapy. Stypoldione, currently being evaluated at the laboratories of Eli Lilly and Company as an anticancer agent, has shown cytotoxicity against several human neoplastic cell lines *in vitro* and *in vivo*. Testing at the National Cancer Institute has shown that the compound also is effective against a specific kind of murine leukemia. Its mechanism of action is only slightly different from, but is complementary to, the mechanism of action of vincristine. Hence, stypoldione has promise as an anticancer drug used in conjunction with other drugs. It is hoped that, using the techniques of biotechnology, researchers will be able to add an antibody to stypoldione that will cause it to bind to a specific cancer protein, ultimately killing cancer cells. Because it inhibits cell division, stypoldione may be useful in treating other kinds of diseases characterized by growing cells, for example parasitic diseases such as schistosomiasis.

Through research on the blood of the horseshoe crab, Dr. G. Sharma *et al.* identified proteins useful for measuring vitamin B_{12} in human fluids.[10] Lack of the vitamin in man can result in pernicious anemia, gastric or intestinal damage, or mental disorders. The reagent currently used for determining vitamin B_{12} costs thousands of dollars per milligram and is not as selective in reaction as the newly-discovered proteins which are expected to cost only a few dollars per milligram. They bind B_{12} with a specificity approaching that of mammalian intrinsic factors, with a binding constant of *ca.* 10^{11} M^{-1}.

Although concentrations of vitamin B_{12} and its analogues, the cobalamins, are extremely low in oceanic waters, many marine organisms are able to satisfy their biological needs for these nutrients by taking them from the sea. Dr. Sharma hypothesized that these organisms accomplish this remarkable feat because their own proteins bind vitamin B_{12} and its analogues. He and his associates confirmed this hypothesis by isolating the binding proteins from horseshoe crabs, clams, and sponges. They conducted detailed studies of the horseshoe crab, *Limulus polyphemus*, for several reasons. First, *Limulus* is a primitive animal and a comparative study of its proteins and those of highly advanced terrestrial animals would aid in revealing evolutionary changes. Second, the horseshoe crab could serve as a model for understanding the mechanisms which facilitate the uptake of B_{12} by cells. Finally, if it is rich in B_{12}-binding proteins, *Limulus* could find an additional use in commerce. *Limulus* plasma is a waste product of the commercial preparation of the clinical reagent lysate, which is widely used to detect bacterial toxins in blood and drugs. Dr. Sharma is now working with a private firm to refine extraction procedures and to develop a test kit that is expected to be used by physicians and clinical chemists. The new reagent also may be important in determining the nutritional role of cobalamins in the primary productivity of the oceans.

GENETIC ENGINEERING

On quite a different tack in biotechnology is the research of Dr. D. Morse of the University of California, Santa Barbara.[11-13] Dr. Morse has shown the potential for adapting modern biochemical and genetic engineering to the control of critical biological processes that limit the efficiency and yield of molluscan production. Dr. Morse found that the swimming larvae of abalone normally are induced to settle from the plankton and metamorphose rapidly to the juvenile form when they contact a chemical signal that is available only at the surfaces of specific red algae. These algae thus normally "recruit" abalone larvae from the plankton. When the abalone larvae encounter these algae in the laboratory, they promptly settle and begin metamorphosis, without any arrest or mortality. Although these red algae clearly satisfy the natural requirements of the abalone larvae for the induction of metamorphosis in nature, the direct use of these algae in aquaculture proved impractical. They grow too slowly for convenient use and, if collected from nature, they are too often contaminated with small predators for reliable use.

Some means of duplicating the natural effect of the algae had to be developed and the chemical inducer normally provided by the algae had to be identified. By column chromatography, Dr. Morse and his associates purified the biochemical substances in these algae which are responsible for the induction of larval abalone settlement and metamorphosis. Biochemical analysis of these purified inducers revealed a family of closely related, active molecules. Of these, the simplest, most potent, and least expensive, proved to be the simple amino acid, γ-aminobutyric acid (GABA); it induces the larvae to settle within minutes. GABA is known to be a potent neurotransmitter or signal molecule in the human brain; this was the first discovery that it also could act to control development in lower animals. Within minutes after the induction of settlement by GABA, the larvae attach to any natural or artificial substrate provided. They begin their life as bottom-dwelling snails and follow their genetically programmed metamorphosis and development to the adult form. Complete metamorphosis is rapidly induced by GABA. No other additions are needed. Internal organ development, including the development and completion of the beating heart, is seen within 60 hours after addition of GABA. In the laboratory, little or no metamorphosis occurs in the absence of GABA; most of the uninduced larvae remain arrested in their development and soon die.

Dr. Morse also showed that hydrogen peroxide induces both male and female abalone to spawn copiously and reliably. The eggs and sperm released in response to peroxide stimulation are fully competent for normal fertilization and development. The method is simple, inexpensive, rapid, and highly reliable. It works because hydrogen peroxide activates the prostaglandin system on which spawning depends.

One of the major problems remaining in the commercial production of abalone is the relatively slow growth of the animal. Here, genetic engineering, as opposed to simple biochemical engineering, can be applied. The California researchers used GABA to induce the start of growth synchronously in order to analyze the hormonal requirements for accelerated growth. From such experiments, they found that very low concentrations of heterologous insulin and growth hormone can accelerate the rate of growth, increase the efficiency of nutrient utilization, and produce greater uniformity of size in juvenile abalones. They also found with sensitive radioimmunoassays that abalones produce these hormones endogenously in very low concentration. Industrial application of these findings will require either the production of large quantities of these hormones inexpensively, or, even better, direct modification of the molluscan genes, so that the animals produce elevated quantities of the hormones themselves. Because molluscs normally make only minute quantities of these hormones, genetic engineering and cloning of the hormone-producing genes will be required, just as these techniques recently have been used for the production of similar hormones for medical purposes, using cloned human genes.

To make possible this industrial application of genetic engineering to mariculture, researchers have begun to clone and amplify the molluscan genes coding for growth-accelerating hormones. DNA obtained in large amounts from abalone sperm by peroxide induction is purified and cut to gene-sized lengths with specific enzymes. The resulting fragments are separated, and those fragments containing genes that code for the production of growth hormones are then identified and purified. Attempts are under way to clone this gene in microorganisms that can be cultured easily.

Extension of this research with GABA and its analogues is relevant to pharmacology. Nearly 50% of the neurons in the human brain and spinal cord, and a number of other specialized receptors, are controlled by the neurotransmitter GABA. As a result, a large proportion of medical prescriptions written in the United States are for agents that act at receptors and sites of uptake for GABA, for control of convulsion, sleep, psychological state, muscle function, degenerative diseases, and other central nervous system functions and disorders. However, the very large number and wide distribution of GABA neurons present in brain and other nervous tissue, and the relatively low selectivity exhibited by the molecules presently available, limit the specificity of therapeutic control and diagnotic labeling now possible. Increased specificity of GABA-mimetic agents is needed to control more selectively and efficiently specific GABA-regulated functions and to minimize undesirable side effects resulting from the multiplicity of sites of action of therapeutic agents now in use. Increased specificity also is needed to take advantage of recently developed non-invasive diagnostic techniques, such as those of external imaging for high-resolution detection and localization of brain and spinal cord dysfunctions.

Dr. Morse recently found that certain marine algae and bacteria produce a previously unsuspected class of GABA-mimetic peptides. In collaboration with investigators at the Beckman City of Hope Medical Research Institute, he found that these short peptides bind very strongly and selectively to GABA receptors from mammalian brain. Because of their strong binding to brain receptors, and the opportunities for multiple and systematic changes in their peptide structures, these novel compounds from marine algae and bacteria represent a new class of GABA-mimetics that may include useful agents for improved specificity of medical diagnosis and treatment. The overall objective of this Sea Grant research is to identify and develop new GABA-mimetic peptides from marine algae and bacteria for improved medical diagnosis and treatment of cranial and other central nervous system disorders.

BIOCHEMICAL ENGINEERING

Researchers at the University of South Alabama and the University of South Carolina have shown that the isolated organic matrices of oyster and clam shells inhibit crystallization of calcium carbonate,[14-16] the major component of scale in industrial equipment such as boilers and evaporators and a component of biofouling on ships and other marine structures. Drs. Sikes and Wheeler have shown that certain synthetic analogues, polyamino acids, act similarly; they are determining the mechanisms of action and seeking to establish practical applications with industrial collaborators. They hypothesize that the findings may also have important applications in treating syndromes or diseases involving calcification, and they and medical collaborators are proceeding toward these applications.

MICROBIOLOGY AND PHYCOLOGY

Plant physiologists at Washington State University have shown that inexpensive treatment of pea and wheat seeds with the marine polymer chitosan, derived from processing wastes of shrimp and crabs, protects seedlings against fungal diseases.[17-19] In studies on 320 acres in eastern Washington they have shown that wheat yields are increased dramatically, up to 20 percent, by the treatment. Professor L. Hadwiger's research group also has determined that chitosan activates specific disease resistance genes in peas. Conversely, when chitosan is applied to pathogenic fungi of plants, gene function is suppressed. It appears that chitosan attaches to and overwhelms the small quantity of DNA in a fungal cell and suppresses its function. Further study of the mechanism of action is under way.

FUTURE DIRECTIONS

Over the next few years the National Sea Grant College Program expects to expand its research in biochemistry, pharmacology, genetic engineering, microbiology, phycology, and biochemical engineering in order to enhance biotechnological development of marine resources. It is expected that basic studies in physiology will be necessary before mass culture and use of marine microorganisms and cells of higher organisms can be applied to exploration of their chemistry and bioactive products. Determination of new mechanisms of biological and pharmacological activity will be important in advancing science and exploiting these products. In the long term, fundamental research in bioreaction, including photobioreaction, biochemical engineering, and polymer chemistry, may offer special opportunities for using marine organisms of many types to provide bulk chemicals, pigments, vitamins, hormones, enzymes, and pharmacologic agents.

I hope these few examples of accomplishment in fundamental research and brief statements on topics for future research will stimulate more scientists in developing marine resources for economic and social benefit.

REFERENCES

1. Bull, A.T.; Holt, G; Lilly, M.D., *Biotechnology: International Trends and Perspectives*. Organisation for Economic Co-Operation and Development, Paris, 1982, p 21.
2. Ibid., p 23.
3. Shapiro, I.S., *Science (Washington, D.C.)*, 1978, *202*, 287.
4. Schmitt, R.W., *Science (Washington, D.C.)*, 1984, *224*, 1206.
5. Tachibana, K.; Scheuer, P.; Tsukitani, Y.; Kikuchi, H.; Van Engen, D.; Clardy, J.; Copichand, Y.; Schmitz, F.J., *J. Am. Chem. Soc.*, 1981, *103*, 2469.
6. Murakami, M.; Oshima, Y.; Yasumoto, T., *Bull. Jpn. Soc. Sci. Fish.*, 1982, *48*, 69.
7. deSilva, E.D.; Scheuer, P.J., *Tetrahedron Lett.*, 1980, 1611.
8. Jacobs, R.S.; Oliver, P.; Langdon, R.; O'Brien, T.; White, S., *Tetrahedron*, 1985, *41*, 981.
9. Gerwick, W.H.; Fenical, W., *J. Org. Chem.*, 1981, *46*, 22.
10. Sharma, G.M.; Shigeura, H.T.; Liu, L.Y.X., *Biochem. Biophys. Res. Commun.*, 1985, *128*, 241.
11. Morse, D.E.; Duncan, H.; Hooker, N.; Morse, A., *Science (Washington, D.C.)*, 1977, *196*, 298.
12. Morse, D.E.; Hooker, N.; Duncan, H.; Jensen, L., *Science (Washington, D.C.)*, 1979, *204*, 407.
13. Morse, D.E., *Aquaculture*, 1984, *39*, 263.
14. Sikes, C.S.; Wheeler, A.P., in *Biomineralization and Biological Metal Accumulation*, Eds. P. Westbrock & E.W. deJong, Reidel Pub. Co., Amsterdam, pp 285-289.
15. Wheeler, A.P.; Sikes, C.S., *Am. Zool.*, 1984, *24*, 933.
16. Sikes, C.S.; Wheeler, A.P., U.S. Patent 4534881, 1985, 16 pp.
17. Hadwiger, L.A.; Fristensky, B.; Riggleman, R.C. in *Chitin, Chitosan, and Related Enzymes*, John P. Zikakis, Ed., Academic Press, New York, NY, 1984, p 291.
18. Walker-Simmons, M.; Jin, D.; West, C.A.; Hadwiger, L.; Ryan, C.A., *Plant Physiol.*, 1984, *76*, 833.
19. Mauch, F.; Hadwiger, L.; Boller, T., *Plant Physiol.*, 1984, *76*, 607.

Morton Collins
DSV Partners, Princeton, New Jersey 08540, U.S.A.

Funding from Private Capital Markets for Basic, Developmental, and Clinical Research

While the challenges of science and the promises of new technology are of greatest concern to most participants in this meeting, the business aspects of marine research, the problems of paying for this wonderful and interesting work, are the responsibility of another group and must occasionally be considered by scientists who worry about being funded or about funding others.

Over the last five years, the "venture capital community" has received substantial media coverage, and venture capitalists have been described as everything from the rock stars of the 80's to the saviors of the world economic system. Neither is a true characterization. For the past several years, business has not been good, and the venture capital community has been quite active in its role of augmenting management in developing companies. This has led to the story about the difference between a dead dog and a dead venture capitalist lying in the road; there are no skid marks near the venture capitalist!

I shall describe here the concept of venture capital, the role usually played by venture capital, and the methods that venture capitalists use, or should use. I shall trace the recent history of the venture capital industry, especially its size and funding, and provide a brief introduction to the organization I manage, DSV Partners. I shall then discuss the investment return expectations of the private capital community and show why they are what they are. Next, a look at the relatively new interest in biotechnology and a quantitative review of progress to date should put the biotechnology funding problem in perspective and lead to some conclusions and forecasts of future trends.

From a historical viewpoint, an early example of venture capital in action is Queen Isabella's investment in Christopher Columbus. Queen Isabella, the venture capitalist, agreed to invest Spain's money, and Columbus, the entrepreneur, agreed to risk his life and reputation in attempting to improve and expand trade with the Far East. The precise nature of the future rewards was unknown; as it turned out, the results were dramatically different from those originally envisioned.

VENTURE CAPITAL

The primary source of support for new high-technology companies is typically venture capital, whose funds usually cover losses during the three to five years between start-up and profit and loss break-even. Once a company achieves profitability, other sources of funding usually become available. Positive cash flow, however, often does not occur for some time after profitability. The balance sheet matters most to bankers and the profit and loss statement is an accountant's fictional attempt to keep score for the company, but it is the cash flow that pays the bills, salaries, and other expenses, literally determining the survival of the company. Indeed, small companies are cash flow-driven, and in the venture capital business happiness is positive cash flow!

Venture capitalists create new businesses or expand and revitalize existing ones by making high-risk, high-reward investments and by assisting the chosen entrepreneurs in developing their businesses. Both the venture capitalist and the entrepreneur work to make the business a long-term operational success. I like to think of this as a partnership--the venture capitalist provides capital and experience, while the entrepreneur contributes creative talent, boundless energy, and hard work.

What is an entrepreneur? The definition given by the *New York Times* on March 25, 1984, in an article entitled "A Pioneer Spirit Sweeps Business" is as follows: "New Entrepreneur--a person, usually under 40, independent and imaginative, who starts a business selling a new product or service in the fast-changing American marketplace; most outstanding examples of the species are in high technology, but they also have profited mightily in cookies, clothing, medical services, etc." There are other definitions; we at DSV view the entrepreneur as the engine that pulls the train up the hill. Entrepreneurs answer to many descriptions, and I cannot define one exactly. I always know, however, when I am in the presence of one.

In order for the venture capitalist to play his partnership role, he must have the time to do so. A rule of thumb in our organization limits each partner to six projects, generally involving six board seats. Most young companies have monthly board meetings, and we usually spend the day of that meeting as well as one additional day per month with the company. Thus, the plan requires two days per month with each of six companies, that is, 144 days per year or 60% of the available time. We actually spend 70-80% of our time working in a partnership role with our companies. It is clear, therefore, that venture capital is principally a business development rather than an investment selection process; investment selection is surely an important first step, but only a first step.

At DSV, investments average *ca.* \$750,000 per company, so that each partner manages approximately \$4.5 million at a time. Overall venture industry statistics--12 investments and \$10 million handled by each partner--indicate the basic cause of problems in the field.

Table I shows the commitments to (investments) and disbursements from the venture capital industry as well as the size of the industry based on capital on hand. Assets remained essentially steady at \$2.5 billion for a decade before dramatic growth began in 1978 and reached a peak during 1983-1984. Assets in 1985 total in excess of \$16 billion. This strong growth is the result of changes in tax and regulatory policy at the Federal level.

DSV PARTNERS

Data Science Ventures (DSV) was formed in 1968 as a privately held venture capital entity to provide capital and management assistance to high-technology companies at a very early stage in their development; because its initial focus was on data processing and communications, it was named DSV. Four organizations have existed thus far--DSV I from 1968 to 1974; DSV II from 1974 to 1981; DSV III, formed in 1981; and DSV IV, formed in 1985. The latter two currently co-invest on a 50/50 basis. The early bias to invest in companies at a very early, often start-up, stage, with substantial involvement in the activities of affiliate companies, has endured.

By 1985 DSV had made 83 investments and its assets exceeded $100 million. Of those investments, 67 (81%) were start-ups, 14 (17%) were second-stage financings, and 2 (2%) were companies at a later stage of their development. While no rigorous statistics exist, this is probably the highest percentage of start-up investments in the industry. All of the companies except one are high-technology companies. Four (5%) are biotechnology companies--The Liposome Company, Markwell Medical Institute, Photec Diagnostics, and SeaPharm.

The Liposome Company is pioneering new techniques of drug delivery through the use of spherical biomembranes called liposomes. Markwell Medical Institute has developed novel techniques for delivering insulin to the human body and is developing associated technology for monitoring serum glucose levels. Photec Diagnostics has developed technology used in new diagnostic systems. SeaPharm is our most recent biotechnology investment.

INVESTMENT RETURNS

Investors of institutional capital (pension, university endowment, and corporate funds, etc.) turn to venture capital as an investment medium because of its superior return over the past two decades, averaging 25-30% compounded annually on a pre-tax basis. This is 15-20% higher than the prevailing inflation rate, that is, a true return of 15-20%. Institutional sources have become the primary suppliers of capital for the venture industry.

Chart I presents a hypothetical distribution of returns in a typical $60 million venture capital portfolio at the end of six years; most venture partnerships last 5-7 years. A total of 16 investments of $2.5 million each were made with the venture firm as the lead investor, and 10 investments of $1 million each were made as co-investments with other venture firms. A cash reserve of $10 million was maintained. The results of the lead and co-investment activities are illustrated, indicating the number of investments and the multiple of cost earned on each. There results, in combination with the cash reserve and the earnings on the cash reserve, produce assets of $287.6 million. Management costs and fees to the General Partners reduce the return to the investors to $236.3 million or a compound annual return of 25.6% on the $60 million investment. The most successful investments in the Chart I portfolio, those with a 20x multiple of cost, correspond, when annualized, to a compound return of 64.8%. This means that a venture investor must believe that a return of at least 60% compound can be achieved on every investment. A return expectation of 50-100% compound is usually employed by the venture industry, the rate required in a given situation being dependent on the perceived level of risk.

Table II illustrates the implications of the lower end of the expectation scale--50% compound annual return. Here, investment requirements of $1, 5, 10, and 25 million are illustrated at 5, 10, and 15 years to show the value that must be achieved by that investment to produce a 50% compound return. The miracle of compound interest is clearly seen in this illustration! Large financial requirements over long time periods must produce dramatic results. In fact, $20 million invested for 15 years must produce $8.8 billion!

Table II also illustrates the difficulty imposed by long time periods and large capital requirements in the building of value in corporate entities. If it is assumed that the investors who provided the initial capital maintain 25% ownership in the company (the remaining 75% owned by management, employees, and other investors) and that biotechnology companies will be valued ultimately in the public market at 1.5-2.5 times annual revenues (the current range for major pharmaceutical companies), then Table II shows the annual revenue levels that must be achieved for a range of investment levels and time periods. Note that an investment as small as $1 million over a period of only 5 years requires that a $15.2 million revenue company be created. A more realistic example is a $5 million investment for 10 years. This requires that a company having revenues of $577 million be created. To date, nothing approximating these results has occurred. It is clearly difficult to finance biotechnology companies with private capital; the capital requirements are too great and the time required to produce revenue and, hence, company value is too long.

FINANCING BIOTECHNOLOGY COMPANIES

The idea of financing biotechnology is very new by any standard; Table III illustrates a few highlights that have led to the current interest. Since it all started in 1973, more than 300 new biotechnology companies have been formed, the majority of those within the last five years. Much of this activity was driven by the apparent success of Genentech, particularly Genentech's success in the public market.

From an equity point of view, the public market has traditionally provided the least costly source of capital for industry, and it is not surprising that the new biotechnology companies focused rapidly on this fact. The public market has requirements, sometimes overlooked in the short term, that need careful consideration. One such requirement for success is the production of an orderly progression of quarterly earnings. The market will "overlook" this for 6-12 months, but rarely longer. Certainly the new biotechnology companies have little chance to produce revenues, much less earnings; hence, it is not surprising that most of this "cheap" capital disappeared quickly. The numbers of small companies that sold stock in the public market are listed in Table IV. Clearly, this activity peaked in 1983, although significant amounts of capital were raised in 1984 and 1985. Some analysts consider July 7, 1983, the date at which the market broke for biotechnology companies; on that date Smith Barney brought AMGEN to the market at $17/share, valuing the company at $300 million. The stock retreated rapidly to $11/share and never recovered. At the time, final negotiations were underway by others to bring Biotechnology General to the market at $25/share, valuing the company at $125 million. That offering was scheduled for mid-July, but Biotechnology General finally came to the market in October 1983 at $13/share and retreated to $7/share within three trading days.

As private and public support for biotechnology companies contracted, massive searches for other financing occurred. Useful methods include government grant and contract funding, research and development partnerships, corporate partnerships, and offshore funding, particularly from Europe and Japan. Each of these techniques has good and bad points, and it is difficult to generalize about which works best in a given situation.

There is, however, good news on the horizon. Some current trends bode well for future financing of biotechnology companies--many companies are turning the corner from losses to profits; sales of monoclonal antibody-based diagnostic products will exceed $200 million in 1985; sales of humulin, the only approved rDNA product, should reach $60 million in 1985; combinant and monoclonal antibody products now in clinical testing and regulatory review have a favorable outlook; and merger and acquisition activity is significant. These developments will reward the courageous and stimulate courage in new investors.

A total of $43.3 million was raised in the public market in 1980, $4.8 million by Enzo Biochem and $38.5 million by Genentech. In 1981, $139.9 million was raised (Cetus, $115.0 million; Generic Systems, 6.6; Hybritech, 13.3; Monoclonal Antibodies, 5.0). For 1982 the total rose to $209.6 million and major corporate investors began to play a role, as shown in Table V. In 1983 $542.1 million was raised for biotechnology. Notwithstanding the collapse of the public market in mid-1983, the total for 1984 was $164.8 million and, through August 31, the 1985 total was $263.1 million. It is interesting that several biotechnology companies retained substantial quantities of cash and, thus, have "staying power" (Table VI).

Reasonably exact data can be obtained concerning money raised in the public market, but that for the private capital market is less exact, even though the venture capital industry maintains a reasonably accurate accounting. Yearly data from 1980 through the first six months of 1985 (Table VII) indicate a total investment of $1,190.6 million over that 5.5-year period, a staggeringly large total for a risky business that did not exist until 1976!

Combined data for the financing of new biotechnology companies (Table VIII) show a surprisingly significant total of $2.6 billion, equivalent to the total assets of the venture capital industry for the decade of the 70's.

CONCLUSIONS AND FUTURE TRENDS

In summary, then, it can be seen that while private capital has provided most of the financing for new biotechnology companies to date, this will not continue. Most biotechnology companies formed in the 1980-1985 period will not remain independent, but the leaders among those companies have developed financial staying power and much of the available investment capital will flow to them. The time and capital required for building a major company based on biotechnology are too great to be sustained by private capital markets. The cost must be shared by government, major multi-national corporations, the public (through participation in the capital markets), and off-balance sheet financing techniques, such as research and development partnerships. New biotechnology projects financed with private capital will focus sharply on near-term products and revenues. The financial success of the "leading" new biotechnology companies will stimulate a new group of private investors, insuring a continuing supply of private capital for less speculative projects.

It is clear that biotechnology holds great promise and has enormous associated costs, largely those imposed by the regulatory system. From the viewpoint of the world of private capital, biotechnology is very different from the technologies funded in the past. New alliances are required to cope with the costs involved and the next decade will, indeed, be interesting!

TABLE I. VENTURE CAPITAL INDUSTRY FUNDING
($ MILLIONS)

Year	New Commitments to Venture Capital	Disbursements	Industry Size
1969	171	450	2,500
1970	97	350	2,500
1971	95	410	2,500
1972	62	425	2,500
1973	56	450	2,500
1974	57	350	2,500
1975	10	250	2,500
1976	50	300	2,700
1977	39	400	3,000
1978	570	550	3,500
1979	319	1,000	4,000
1980	900	1,100	4,500
1981	1,300	1,400	5,800
1982	1,800	1,800	7,600
1983	4,500	2,800	12,100
1984	4,200	3,000	16,300
1985 (6/30)	1,300	3,000	17,600

CHART I. HYPOTHETICAL DISTRIBUTION OF RETURNS
$60 MILLION VENTURE CAPITAL FUND
SIX YEARS

Portfolio Investments	($ Millions)
16 Lead Investments	40.0
10 Co-Investments	10.0
Cash Reserve	10.0
Total	60.0

Lead Investments

Number	Multiple	Annual Return(%)	Amount
2	20X	64.8	100.0
3	10X	46.8	75.0
3	5X	30.8	37.5
3	2X	12.2	15.0
3	1X	0	7.5
2	0X	0	0.0
			235.0

Co-Investments

Number	Multiple	Annual Return(%)	Amount
1	10X	46.8	10.0
4	5X	30.8	20.0
4	1X	0	4.0
1	0X	0	0.0
			34.0

Cash ($10 Million at 10%/year)	17.7
Total	287.6
Cost of Management (2%/year)	7.2
General Partners Share of Profits (20%)	44.1
Return to Investors	236.3

Compound Annual Investment Return = 25.6%

TABLE II. REQUIRED INVESTMENT VALUE[a]

Initial Capital Requirement ($ Millions)	Value of Investment[a] ($ Millions)			Annual Revenue Requirement[b] ($ Millions)		
	5 Years	10 Years	15 Years	5 Years	10 Years	15 Years
1.0	7.6	57.7	437.9	15.2	115.4	875.8
5.0	38.0	288.5	2,189.5	76.0	577.0	4,379.0
10.0	76.0	577.0	4,379.0	152.0	1,154.0	8,758.0
20.0	152.0	1,154.0	8,758.0	304.0	2,308.0	17,516.0

[a]Annual return requirement, 50%. [b]Assumptions: 1) initial investors retain 25% ownership; 2) biotechnology companies valued at 1.5-2.5 X annual revenues.

TABLE III. COMMERCIALIZATION OF BIOTECHNOLOGY

Year	Event
1973	First gene cloned
1974	First expression of a gene cloned from a different species in bacteria
1975	First hybridoma created
1976	Genentech formed
1980	U.S. Supreme Court decision on the patentability of microorganisms
	Initial public offering of Genentech
1981	First monoclonal antibody approved for use in the United States
	Initial public offering of Cetus
	80+ New biotechnology firms formed
1982	First genetically engineered product (Insulin) approved for use
	First R&D Partnership formed for funding clinical trials
1983	First plant gene expressed in a plant of a different species
	$500+ Million raised in U.S. public market by biotechnology companies
	SeaPharm formed
1984	R&D Partnerships totaling $200+ Million formed

TABLE IV. PUBLIC MARKET - SMALL COMPANIES NEW ISSUES

Year	Number of Companies	Capital Raised ($Million)
1968	358	745
1969	698	1,367
1970	198	375
1971	248	551
1972	409	896
1973	69	160
1974	9	16
1975	4	16
1976	29	145
1977	30	118
1978	37	206
1979	73	368
1980	185	1,306
1981	392	2,646
1982	153	1,130
1983	611	5,740
1984	266	1,680
1985 (8/31)	156	1,150

TABLE V. PUBLIC BIOTECHNOLOGY FINANCINGS (1982-1985)

Company	Corporate Investor	Amount ($ Million) 1982	1983	1984	1985
Advanced Genetic Systems			11.3		
Agracetus					10.0
Amgen			42.3		
Applied Biosystems			19.2	16.9	
" "	Becton Dickinson				18.4
Biogen			63.3	28.0	
Bio-Response			17.4		
BioTechnica International			7.7		
"	Seagram				4.4
Bio-Technology General			10.4		
California Biotechnology			12.0		
"	American Home Products				12.0
Cambridge BioSciences			5.5		
Centocor		23.1		5.0	23.1
Cetus			75.0		
Chiron			19.2		
Collaborative Research		14.3	16.8		
Cooper Biomedical			30.3		
Damon Biotech			40.8		
DNA Plant Technology				14.5	
Enzo Biochem	Johnson & Johnson	14.0			
Genentech		55.6	32.2		51.8
Genentech					31.6
Genentech	Boerhinger Ingelheim				40.0
Genentech	Corning Glass	5.0	5.0		
Genentech	Corning Glass		10.5		
Genentech	Swedish Consortium	20.0			
Genetic Systems			21.7		17.0
Genetic Systems (pending)	Syntex				40.0

Table V (cont.)

Company	Corporate Investor	Amount ($ Million) 1982	1983	1984	1985
Genexc		19.0	24.6		
Hybritech		36.9		70.0	
Hybritech		6.5			
ICN Pharm./Viratek	Eastman Kodak			8.4	
Immunex			18.2		
Integrated Genetics			20.8		
Kirin-Amgen	Kirin Brewing			12.0	
Molecular Genetics		4.1	20.5		
Molecular Genetics		11.1			
Molecular Genetics	Martin Marietta		9.7		
Monoclonal Antibodies			8.2		
Oncogen	Bristol-Myers				12.8
Ribi ImmunoChem					12.0
	Total	$209.6	$542.1	$164.8	$263.1

TABLE VI. CASH HELD BY PUBLIC BIOTECHNOLOGY COMPANIES

Company	Amount ($ Million)
Genentech	101
Genetic Systems (Pending Syntex)	88
Cetus	85
Biogen	64
Applied Biosystems	56
	394
All Others	238
Total	632

TABLE VII. VENTURE CAPITAL - BIOTECHNOLOGY INVESTMENTS

Year	Disbursements ($ Million)	Biotech ($ Million)	% of Disbursed Funds
1980	1,100	88.0	8.0
1981	1,400	154.0	11.0
1982	1,800	478.8	11.2
1983	2,800	310.8	11.1
1984	3,000	63.0	2.1
1985 (6/30)	3,000	96.0	3.2
Total		1,190.6	

TABLE VIII. TOTAL CAPITAL RAISED BY NEW BIOTECHNOLOGY COMPANIES (1980-1985)

Financing Method	Total ($ Million)
Venture Capital	1,190.6
Public Equity	769.1
Corporate Equity	238.6
R&D Partnerships	355.1
Total	2,553.4